To Barbara Fitzg

in grateful appreciation

Dick Edlich

Medicine's Deadly Dust

A Surgeon's Wake-up Call to Society

About The Author

Richard F. Edlich, M.D., Ph.D., is a world-renowned authority on surgical wound healing and infection. He is a Distinguished Professor of Plastic Surgery and Biomedical Engineering at the University of Virginia School of Medicine, where his research laboratory has devised surgical techniques that allow wounds to heal without infection and with the most aesthetically pleasing scar. In his earlier studies, he devised long intestinal tubes that decompressed the intestine without surgical intervention. His gastric lavage kit for cleansing the stomach is used throughout the world. His pioneering clinical studies of endoscopy of the stomach led to the development of nonoperative percutaneous gastrotomy. As a specialist in research on the development and prevention of intestinal adhesions, as well as on the biology of wound repair and infection, he has published six books and more than 600 scientific articles.

Dr. Edlich is the recipient of the highest academic honor at the University of Virginia, the Thomas Jefferson Award. In addition, endowments have been established for the annual Richard F. Edlich Lecture, the Richard F. Edlich Chair in Surgical Research, and the Richard F. Edlich University of Virginia Medical Student Research Award.

Medicine's Deadly Dust
A Surgeon's Wake-up Call to Society

Richard F. Edlich, M.D., Ph.D.
with Julia A. Woods and Mary Jude Cox

VANDAMERE
PRESS

Published by
Vandamere Press
P.O. Box 5243
Arlington, VA 22205

Copyright 1997
Vandamere Press

ISBN 0-918339-45-6

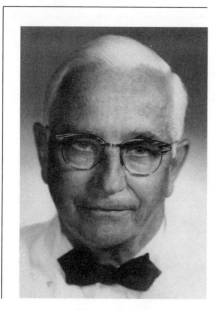

Dr. Owen H. Wangensteen

I have dedicated Medicine's Deadly Dust, *to my esteemed mentor, colleague, and friend, Dr. Owen Harding Wangensteen, who is recognized as the most important surgeon-educator in the United States during the 20th century. On January 13, 1981, the teacher of surgical teachers, Dr. Owen Wangensteen, died. His success as a teacher, as judged by the number and level of academic full-time appointments filled by his students speaks for itself: 38 department chairmen; 31 division heads; 72 directors of training programs; 110 full professors; and 18 associate professors.*

Dr. Wangensteen was always concerned that many surgeons used outdated surgical techniques that endangered their patients. I have written Medicine's Deadly Dust *to educate the public about several important aspects of contemporary healthcare excellence, and to awaken society to new concepts of surgical care that are important in preventing avoidable complications. With this knowledge, the patient can become a vital partner in modern healthcare.*

Acknowledgements

At the University of Virginia School of Medicine, my research has been a multidisciplinary effort, involving distinguished scientists who formed the foundation for a strong and productive research laboratory. It is a duteous pleasure to acknowledge Dr. George T. Rodeheaver, research professor of plastic surgery, and Dr. John G. Thacker, professor of mechanical and aerospace engineering, who have been my partners in research programs for the last 25 years. This research also involved literally hundreds of undergraduate students, medical students, postdoctoral fellows, and residents. In our academic journey, we realize that the contribution of our intellectual progeny will far exceed our own, a reward that is the essence of teaching. I have included a section in the appendix of the book that acknowledges every student and faculty member who has worked in our research laboratory (Appendix A). Their enormous scientific discoveries provided a fertile academic environment that allowed us to study the deadly dust in medicine.

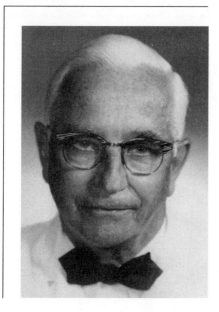

Dr. Owen H. Wangensteen

I have dedicated Medicine's Deadly Dust, *to my esteemed mentor, colleague, and friend, Dr. Owen Harding Wangensteen, who is recognized as the most important surgeon-educator in the United States during the 20th century. On January 13, 1981, the teacher of surgical teachers, Dr. Owen Wangensteen, died. His success as a teacher, as judged by the number and level of academic full-time appointments filled by his students speaks for itself: 38 department chairmen; 31 division heads; 72 directors of training programs; 110 full professors; and 18 associate professors.*

Dr. Wangensteen was always concerned that many surgeons used outdated surgical techniques that endangered their patients. I have written Medicine's Deadly Dust *to educate the public about several important aspects of contemporary healthcare excellence, and to awaken society to new concepts of surgical care that are important in preventing avoidable complications. With this knowledge, the patient can become a vital partner in modern healthcare.*

Acknowledgements

At the University of Virginia School of Medicine, my research has been a multidisciplinary effort, involving distinguished scientists who formed the foundation for a strong and productive research laboratory. It is a duteous pleasure to acknowledge Dr. George T. Rodeheaver, research professor of plastic surgery, and Dr. John G. Thacker, professor of mechanical and aerospace engineering, who have been my partners in research programs for the last 25 years. This research also involved literally hundreds of undergraduate students, medical students, postdoctoral fellows, and residents. In our academic journey, we realize that the contribution of our intellectual progeny will far exceed our own, a reward that is the essence of teaching. I have included a section in the appendix of the book that acknowledges every student and faculty member who has worked in our research laboratory (Appendix A). Their enormous scientific discoveries provided a fertile academic environment that allowed us to study the deadly dust in medicine.

The unsuspecting individuals who are being injured daily by medicine's deadly dust will first seek the advice and counsel of their treating physicians regarding their illnesses. When their physicians fail to identify the cause of their illnesses, patients usually ask for second opinions from other clinicians.

Many patients will ultimately learn that their injuries due to medicine's deadly dust could have been easily prevented, a realization that is resulting in increasing numbers of lawsuits. In my discussion of a guide for malpractice and consumer product litigation regarding medicine's deadly dust, I sought the advice of the respected attorney, Catherine J. Furay in Madison, Wisconsin.

It is important to point out that two of our most gifted students played a key role in writing this book. Julia Woods, an important member of our research team, has made numerous innovative, scientific contributions that have provided a more accurate picture of the deadly dust's damaging effect on human tissue. Her investigative talents will continue to be recognized as she pursues a successful career in academic plastic surgery. My esteemed colleague, Mary Jude Cox, has made pioneering research contributions in studies of the biomechanical performance of surgical gloves during the last seven years. Her heart is set on a career in academic ophthalmic surgery, a specialty that is indeed fortunate to gain the benefits of her creative mind. I know that both Julia and Mary Jude will serve as wonderful role models for young women considering a career in academic medicine.

In addition, I have always recognized the generous donors who have thoughtfully supported our research program. Their generous gifts have been instrumental in allowing our laboratory to grow and bring technologic advances to surgery. During the last 30 years, I have contacted friends of our laboratory and updated them on our progress. Throughout my career, I have developed close personal friendships with these generous supporters, who continue to encourage us to pursue our dreams. I have identified the names of these generous donors in another appendix of the book (Appendix B).

I want to especially acknowledge Dr. Raymond F. Morgan, Chairman of the Department of Plastic Surgery at the University of Virginia School of Medicine, who has valiantly supported the development of our comprehensive research program that has brought scientific advances to the patient's bedside.

Richard F. Edlich, M.D., Ph.D.

Contents

Foreword

... from the perspective of a teacher of surgery

by Stuart S. Howards, M.D.

Medicine's deadly dusts and life-threatening latex allergy are critical public health issues, which have received surprisingly little attention from the scientific or lay press. With the publication of *Medicine's Deadly Dust*, Richard F. Edlich, M.D., Ph.D., has brought this serious topic to the forefront with a careful and thoughtful exploration of the issues.

As he points out in the introduction of the book, Dr. Edlich had an early and tragic awakening to the subject of intestinal obstruction. At the age of 11, watching his mother suffer, he

Dr. Stuart S. Howards, Professor of Urology and Physiology, is an internationally renowned specialist in pediatric urology and male infertility. He is the Editor of the Investigative Section of the *Journal of Urology*. He is one of the editors of a scholarly textbook of urology, *Adult and Pediatric Urology*, that is read by surgeons and urologists throughout the world. He is the recipient of the Hugh Hampton Young Award and the Russell Scott Award from the American Urologic Association.

could not guess that he would grow up to dedicate 30 years of medical research to investigating the causes of, and strategies to eliminate, this complication that often follows abdominal surgery. Few physicians are as uniquely qualified to write a book on this subject as Dr. Edlich. His academic credentials are impeccable, and his career is studded with remarkable achievements that reach far beyond the field of plastic surgery. Dr. Edlich received a Ford Foundation Scholarship for early admission to college at 15 years of age. He progressed rapidly through the educational system to graduate from medical school 4 years before his contemporaries at the remarkable age of 22. Dr. Edlich went to work with Dr. Owen H. Wangensteen, Professor and Chairman of the Department of Surgery at the University of Minnesota. Dr. Wangensteen was a gifted and revered teacher who trained a long list of academic general surgeons. In 1971, Dr. Edlich joined the Department of Plastic Surgery at the University of Virginia in Charlottesville, Virginia. It is there that our paths crossed. I came to know him as a friend and to admire his integrity, his keen probing mind, and his dogged determination to see a problem through to solution.

Dr. Edlich's interests have often distinguished him from his peers. He chose to turn down offers to be Chairman of Plastic Surgery or General Surgery, which could have brought him greater status and income. He preferred, instead, to devote himself to research, teaching, and excellence in patient care. During his tenure at the University of Virginia, Dr. Edlich has been a mentor to many young doctors. The medical students have listened to his outstanding lectures and chosen to honor him year after year. His peers have also recognized Dr. Edlich's achievements through the Richard F. Edlich Burn Lecture and the Richard F. Edlich Chair in Plastic Surgical Research at the University of Virginia. Dr. Edlich has held a joint appointment in Biomedical Engineering since 1978.

Above and beyond his dedication to the ideals of medicine, beyond his scholarship, and his 600 publications, Dr. Edlich is unique because of his creative and courageous thinking. He has blazed a trail in the development of surgical products and in the cooperative interaction of academic physicians with industry. He has repeatedly ventured where others might fear to tread. Long before Emergency Medicine was popular or became a major specialty, Dr. Edlich put his energy into setting up and coordinating emergency medical services to benefit the University of Virginia and the rest of the state. He is clearly a pioneer in the field.

Dr. Edlich was also a driving force in a major effort to set up the University of Virginia Burn Center where he served as director. Few physicians have the patience or the selflessness to deal with the tragic consequences of major burns. In addition to those demands, Dr. Edlich continued to maintain a large practice in plastic surgery and to oversee an extensive research facility devoted to wound care and healing. He found time to direct the Life-Support Learning Center at the University and he codirected the Emergency Nurse Practitioner Training Program and the National Crisis Center for the Deaf.

It is a pleasure to recommend this interesting and readable text on an important public health issue. Dr. Edlich provides the lay reader and the healthcare professional with unique insights into the problem of medicine's deadly dust and latex allergy. He has chosen to incorporate the history of five patients into the text, drawing the reader to the significance of these problems at a very human level. His recommendations for a solution are logical and backed by scientific data not always found in texts dealing with environmental and public health issues. We are presented with the important results of the change to powder-free gloves at the Brigham and Women's Hospital in Boston, and the experience at the Mayo Clinic using powder-free sterile gloves with low levels of latex allergens as a cost-effective alternative.

Finally, although it may not be popular with other physicians, Dr. Edlich provides an appendix with a guide for malpractice and consumer product litigation. He proposes a common sense, cost-effective solution that could change the surgical environment in operating rooms across the country, saving a significant group of patients from serious postsurgical complications.

Stuart S. Howards, M.D.
Professor of Urology
University of Virginia Medical School
Charlottesville, Virginia

. . . from the perspective of a disability rights attorney

by Evan J. Kemp, Jr.

I firmly believe that, given the proper products, necessary resources, and adequate information, consumers, including those with disabilities and chronic health conditions, are capable of making informed decisions about their safety and health. Unfortunately, consumers are frequently denied the opportunities to make such decisions.

In particular, consumers have not been given access to information about the dangers inherent in medical products, such as surgical gloves containing latex and dangerous powders. Through his own experience and other real-life stories, renowned plastic surgeon, Dr. Richard Edlich, rectifies this situation. In his book, *Medicine's Deadly Dust,* he provides a

Formerly Chairman of the U.S. Equal Employment Opportunity Commission, Evan J. Kemp, Jr., is one of the authors of the Americans With Disabilities Act. He is currently the Chairman of Evan Kemp Associates, Inc., which provides news, information, and products and services to people with disabilities and chronic health conditions so that they may make informed choices and lead active and independent lives.

believably detailed account of a dangerous health issue—the use of medical products that are laced with irritating and potentially deadly dust in the health care environment. Because of universal precautions to protect hospital workers from exposure to blood and bodily fluids, the use of medical products, such as latex gloves, has greatly increased as has the hated latex allergies—especially among health care professionals. This increased risk to healthcare professionals, in turn, has directed attention to the dangers caused by exposure to massive amounts of these irritating powders. Most of the public, however, is still unaware of the dangers that even small amounts of this deadly dust can cause.

Now, for the first time, a highly respected medical professional speaks up and brings this issue to the public's attention. In *Medicine's Deadly Dust*, Dr. Edlich warns that the situation is far more serious, dangerous, and costly than anyone realizes. In his book, Dr. Edlich explains that the serious health risks associated with these powders are only superficially understood in the medical community and virtually unknown in the lay world. While powder-free gloves are readily available, the manufacture and use of powdered surgical gloves continue to flourish. Only a few hospitals and individual practitioners are beginning to insist on powder-free products to avoid the risks to both patients and health care workers.

Medicine's Deadly Dust traces the use of different powders in surgical gloves from the 1800s to the present. Dr. Edlich draws clear links between serious tissue healing complications that have historically gone unexplained and dust from surgical gloves. When some surgical tissue is reexamined, large inflammatory nodules and thick binding internal scars or adhesions are frequently found to contain clumps of powder from surgical gloves. People who react to these powders on surgical gloves experience adhesions that can cause unbearable pain and cramping. Frequently, adhesion lysis surgery is performed to reduce intestinal adhesions. The same surgical procedure often must be repeated many times because, with each successive surgery, the medical personnel using powdered gloves deposit more irritating powder into the unsuspecting patient's body cavity. The fresh powder deposits form new adhesions that, in turn, require more surgery. It can be a never-ending, dangerously vicious cycle. These surgical procedures are performed too frequently and at a tremendous cost. In 1988, for example, **281,982** *hospital admissions* in the United States were for adhesion breakdown surgery. The estimated annual cost of these hospital procedures is almost $1.2 billion, but the dollar cost pales in comparison to the human cost.

Between 1988 and 1995, the FDA received reports of 23 deaths from "allergic reactions" related to the use of medical products containing latex. Inflammatory responses to latex allergens, such as those found on the powders in the gloves, can include swelling of the head and neck and severe shortness of breath. If left untreated and without quick emergency care, these allergic responses can result in anaphylactic shock, a state of collapse with complete airway obstruction and ultimately death. The life-threatening anaphylactic response appears within minutes after exposure to latex in allergic individuals. Exposure to latex during surgery is the route most often associated with deadly anaphylactic reactions. People with disabilities and chronic health conditions who encounter a significant number of latex medical products, such as tubes, syringes and catheters, are especially at high risk for developing a life-threatening latex allergy.

Dr. Edlich reveals the failure of the Food and Drug Administration (FDA) to take a leadership role in regulating the use of powder in gloves. Current regulations require examination of gloves with respect to several characteristics such as sterility, size and presence of holes. However, the FDA does not prohibit the deadly dust, despite reports documenting its dangers.

I applaud Dr. Edlich for his professional dedication and the valuable public service he performs with this book. It not only warns the public about these dangerous products, but also provides information about product liability issues and litigation procedures. I believe that an informed consumer can advocate change, and Dr. Edlich's knowledgeable and informative book gives consumers the tools. Armed with the information contained in Dr. Edlich's book, and for their own protection, consumers, especially those facing elective surgery, should

- question physicians about the measures they have taken to limit latex exposure and eliminate the deadly dust from products used in their practice
- contact hospital administrators and insist that they purchase only powder-free surgical gloves
- insist that hospitals maintain latex-free operating suites
- demand that medical professionals stop using products containing high levels of latex allergens and harmful powders.

For anyone facing elective surgery or for those who regularly use products containing latex, either personally or professionally, *Medicine's Deadly Dust* contains valuable information that can save lives.

Evan J. Kemp, Jr.
Washington, D.C.
January 1997

Medicine's Deadly Dust

A Surgeon's Wake-up Call to Society

Introduction

"Each of us has many potential selves. It is within the power of most of us to decide what manner of man and physician we shall be."

Dr. Owen H. Wangensteen

The trials and tribulations of childhood can have a profound impact on our lives. In some cases, they become a guide for our journeys through life. When I was 11 years old, my mother had abdominal surgery for a large ovarian cyst. After surgery we celebrated the good news about the benign nature of the cyst, but we had no idea that this surgery was just the beginning of a devastating cycle of illness caused by recurrent intestinal obstruction.

During the next four years, she had repeated attacks of intestinal obstruction caused by thin fibrous strands of tissue (adhesions) that compressed her bowels. I can distinctly remember her complaints of intermittent episodes of abdominal pain that were not localized to any region of her abdomen. She would depart from the family and go quickly to the bathroom to shield her children from the miseries of her illness. I can still hear her repeated retching that emptied fluid and air from her stomach. I would call my father, a doctor, hoping that he would rescue her from her plight and allow her to

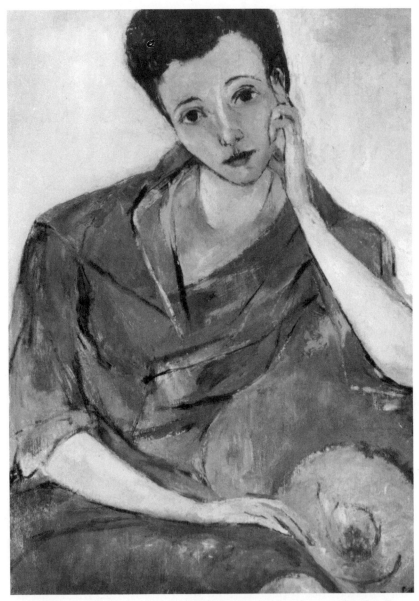

A portrait of my mother, Virginia Edlich, painted by the noted artist, Franz Kline. Kline captures a pensive moment in her life at a time when she courageously struggled with recurrent bouts of intestinal obstruction.

remain at home. The situation, however, was always the same: the emergency medical technician would arrive to gently lift her onto a stretcher and transfer her by ambulance to the hospital.

After arriving at the hospital, we would all join in the waiting game to see if surgery was necessary to relieve my mother's intestinal obstruction. With the nasogastric tube positioned in her nasal canal, I would watch the evacuation of fluids from her stomach being collected in a large transparent container. While this removal of nasogastric fluids from her stomach visibly reduced her abdominal bloating, the development of recurrent pain would be a sign that she would have to return to surgery and thus be absent from home for at least three weeks.

Her frequent hospitalizations left my father to nurture and support my brothers and me. My father's graphic discussions of her surgical treatment were intended to provide us with hope for her quick recovery without need for further surgical treatments. He described to us the adhesions in her abdominal cavity that compressed and obstructed her bowel. After the surgeons cut the adhesive bands of tissue, relieving the obstruction, he said that they washed her abdominal cavity with large amounts of saltwater to remove any material that would be causing these adhesions. Naively, I never questioned my father about the cause for these adhesions, assuming that neither he nor the surgeons had a clear understanding of why these adhesions developed in her abdominal cavity and eventually compressed the bowel, causing the obstruction.

Because of my father's love for his wife as well as his respect for medicine, he always believed that each operative procedure would solve her nightmare. Consequently, he remained optimistic and provided convincing arguments for our family's return to peace and harmony. Despite my father's assurances, I then felt considerable uncertainty and despair about my mother's illness. It was this fear and feeling of helplessness that provided my career direction.

I received a Ford Foundation scholarship for early admission to college at the age of 15, providing me with an opportunity to escape from home, where I was paralyzed by fear of my mother's next possible hospitalization. I entered Lafayette College with mixed emotions. While I was honored to be accepted into a pioneering educational program for gifted students, I also felt enormous guilt in abandoning my mother, realizing that I was not able to help her. My profound sadness coupled with this guilt were the major reasons for my pursuit of studies in intestinal obstruction during the last 30 years.

By 1958, I had accelerated my educational programs so rapidly that I never graduated from high school or college. At age 18, I began my medical school education at the New York University College of Medicine. By 1962, I was 22 years old and my heart was set on a career in academic medicine. Because the door of the Department of Surgery at the University of Minnesota was open to all aspiring residents interested in a career in teaching, I decided to immerse myself in that academic village. Dr. Owen Wangensteen, who is recognized as the greatest teacher of surgery of the last century, was the Chairman of the Department. His major academic objective was to create an atmosphere that was friendly to learning, for scholars who dreamed of changing the world.

One of Dr. Wangensteen's most important contributions to surgery were his studies of intestinal obstruction. These studies resulted in revolutionary clinical advances. He defined the criteria for the early diagnosis of intestinal obstruction with the aid of a stethoscope and X-ray examination. Moreover, he discovered that suction with a nasal catheter extending to the stomach could relieve the obstruction as effectively as surgery. This same tube was used to remove the air and fluid from my mother's obstructed intestine. His proposed nonoperative treatment of intestinal obstruction constituted a revolutionary advance in surgery.

By the time I arrived at Dr. Wangensteen's academic village in 1963, he had dramatically reduced the death rate from intestinal obstruction from 60 percent to 6 percent. Dr. Wangensteen believed that the death rate from acute intestinal obstruction could be reduced even further if the bowel could be decompressed by a long intestinal tube. In an effort to achieve this goal, he trained his surgical residents to use long intestinal tubes as part of the immediate treatment of acute intestinal obstruction. His conservative management of acute intestinal obstruction became essentially a team effort led by surgical residents. Success with conservative decompression demanded a team of enthusiastic and experienced residents who were able to use nasogastric tubes as well as longer intestinal tubes skillfully through patients' nasal canals into their stomachs and small intestines. Dr. Wangensteen encouraged each resident to take the lead in this field. I joined the team! I developed a directional fingerlike balloon at the end of the tube that facilitated passing this tube through the stomach into the small intestine. He believed that my new intestinal tube extended the techniques of intestinal intubation that made it possible to decompress the small bowel effectively, prior to operation without needing surgery.

Because Dr. Wangensteen viewed himself as a "plumber of the digestive tract," I anticipated that he would involve me in his clinical and experimental research studies of the gastrointestinal system, which would ultimately lead me to an academic career in general surgery. He welcomed all my suggestions, especially those that shed light on the gastrointestinal tract. Without hesitation, he purchased flexible fiberoptic endoscopes used to to visualize a dangerous bleeding site within the stomach and esophagus. As a third-year resident, I was the first individual to perform endoscopy of

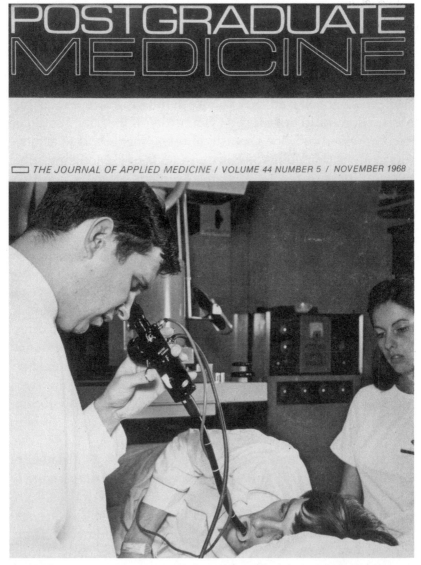

POSTGRADUATE MEDICINE

THE JOURNAL OF APPLIED MEDICINE / VOLUME 44 NUMBER 5 / NOVEMBER 1968

A photograph on the cover of the journal, *Postgraduate Medicine,* features the author performing endoscopic examination of the esophagus and the stomach during his surgical residency.

the esophagus and stomach at the University of Minnesota Health Sciences Center in 1967. In my initial clinical trials with these instruments, it became readily apparent that removal of blood clots from the patient's stomach prior to endoscopy was mandatory to permit visualization of the bleeding site. A thick-walled rubber tube was inadequate for this task because its small internal diameter became obstructed by blood clots. I quickly resolved this problem by designing a disposable, transparent, thin-walled gastric tube and syringe that allowed rapid and complete removal of blood clots from the stomach.

The use of fiberoptic endoscopy in our laboratory had other immediate clinical applications. During endoscopy, the stomach becomes filled with air, which pushes the front wall of the stomach against the inner lining of the abdominal cavity. In a darkened room, the endoscopic light source reveals the site of contact between the stomach and the abdominal wall, allowing the identification of an appropriate site for an incision. This incision then provides ready access for the passage of a feeding tube through the abdominal and stomach walls into the stomach cavity, avoiding the need for major surgery. The practicality of this method was tested and demonstrated on human cadavers, and subsequently was performed on an elderly, critically ill patient with the use of local anesthesia. This procedure has since been modified by other physicians using a technique in which a permanent feeding tube is passed using the fiberoptic endoscope.

Robert Goodale, coresident and friend, later used our flexible fiberoptic endoscope to advance the long intestinal tube through the stomach and into the small intestine. This entire procedure, which takes less than 15 minutes, is reliable and relatively easy when performed by skilled and trained physicians like Bob Goodale.

While Dr. Wangensteen was always pleased with the results of our efforts to treat patients with intestinal obstruction, he realized that prevention of intestinal obstruction is a far superior goal. In his classic textbook, *Intestinal Obstruction,** Dr. Wangensteen emphasized the technical features and operations that predisposed to adhesion formation. He felt that trauma was an important irritant. He used the term," traumatic surgery," facetiously to describe the harmful effects of poor surgical technique. He discouraged the use of highly reactive suture materials, such as chromic catgut, as well as sutures with a wide diameter.

Earlier in his surgical career, Dr. Wangensteen had pointed out that Dr. William Antopol from Bayonne Hospital in Bayonne, New Jersey, presented findings at the New York Pathologic Society on October 8, 1931, that indicated the clinical significance of inflammatory reactions caused by surgical glove dusting powders, medicine's deadly dust. Dr. Antopol later published these important findings in the journal, *Archives of Pathology*, in 1933, the first report to alert surgeons that talcum powder on surgical gloves could produce non-cancerous inflammatory nodules that could be confused with cancers. Additional research during Dr. Wangensteen's surgical carreer provided further insight into the causes of intestinal adhesions. In 1943, Dr. William McKee German, from the University of Cincinnati Department of Pathology, found experimental evidence in animals to indicate that talcum powder, then used by most surgeons to ease glove donning, severely irritated tissues and provoked adhesions in the abdominal cavity. Dr. Wangensteen commented that all surgeons had seen talc granulomas causing intestinal obstruction. In 1947, Dr. Edwin Partridge Lehman, Professor and Chairman of Surgery and Gynecology at the University of

---

* For source information, readers should consult the Reference Notes section at the end of the book. Entries are organized by chapter and arranged alphabetically for ease of reference by the reader.

Virginia, was the first to suggest replacing the talcum powder with a starch powder. Dr. Lehman recommended this change, in part, because talcum powder was not absorbed into the body when it was left in the abdominal cavity, causing numerous problems. In contrast, the starch was slowly absorbed when left in the body. Surgeons initially thought that the use of the absorbable cornstarch promoted by Dr. Lehman was complication-free and a vast improvement over the use of talcum powder. Five years later, Dr. C. Marshall Lee, Jr., from the University of Cincinnati, reported disturbing findings in abdominal wounds in dogs following the use of starch powder in surgery. When the wounds were infected, the presence of cornstarch promoted adhesion formation. Dr. Lee pointed out that, even in clean wounds, starch powder behaved as an irritating substance until it was completely absorbed. At the end of his classic report, Dr. Lee emphasized: "Every possible precaution should be taken to prevent powder contamination of open wounds or serosal surfaces, and no powder is so 'safe' that it can be carelessly used."

Based on these early studies Dr. Wangensteen warned surgeons that they should wash away any trace of starch powder remaining on the outside of rubber gloves before starting an operation. In 1954, Clarence Dennis, one of his protegés, emphasized the importance of washing off glove powder with two large wet sponges. Dennis felt that washing the gloved hand in a basin was inadequate to remove the powder.

Later, during the late 1960s, while I was intubating, illuminating, and penetrating the gastrointestinal tract, Dr. Wangensteen was searching for and collecting information relating to the historical management of wounds in times of peace and war. He conjured up an enormous number of innovative ideas in wound repair that would prevent infection. After Dr. Wangensteen shared these ideas with me, I agreed with him that wound healing should become the major new focus of my research efforts. Obediently I left the portals of the intestinal tract to become a surgeon who focused research on the healing of wounds and wound infection. This change in the direction of my research program was the beginning of my personal odyssey in research that has continued without interruption for nearly 30 years.

Near the end of my general surgical residency, Dr. Wangensteen suggested that I pursue a career in academic plastic surgery, a clinical specialty devoted to the study of the biology of wound repair and infection. He carefully orchestrated my move from general surgery to plastic surgery. He contacted Dr. Milton Edgerton, one of the most respected academic plastic surgeons in our country, and recommended me for a position in his residency at the University of Virginia School of Medicine. Dr. Wangensteen suggested that I receive a faculty appointment, which would enable me to be the recipient of his research grant. He asked that the University of Virginia School of Medicine give me adequate research space for the two laboratory technicians and research equipment that would accompany me to Virginia. Realizing the financial hardship that I would be facing during my ninth and tenth years of residency training (1971-1973), he also requested that my salary be supplemented above that of the plastic surgery residents.

At the University of Virginia School of Medicine, my research was a multidisciplinary effort, involving distinguished scientists who formed the foundation for a strong and productive research laboratory. The results of our research have greatly surpassed our expectations. We have identified numerous innovative surgical techniques that prevent infection as well as adhesion formation. These surgical techniques have been incorporated into a teaching curriculum that is being used to teach surgeons and physicians throughout the world. I believe that surgery is on the threshold of a new horizon in which wounds can be repaired without infection and adhesions and with the most aesthetically pleasing scar. Despite the overwhelming evidence for the use of these new innovative approaches in surgery, many surgeons are reluctant to change, being guided by ritual practice rather than scientific discipline. Consequently, I am writing this book to alert the public about the deadly dust of medicine, so that the surgeon and patient can become educated champions for abandoning the use of this dangerous powder.

CHAPTER ONE

Random Happenings

"It was a crack in the door that emitted enough light to permit resolution of the problem in an effective manner. How long it takes to find the crack!"

Dr. Owen H. Wangensteen

To introduce the reader to the problems associated with medicine's deadly dusts in the environment, I have selected five cases who experienced a wide variety of unexplained complications during their medical care. Reports of each of these five patients' stories actually appeared in the medical literature. In an effort to maintain patient privacy, the identifying characteristics of the hospitals, doctors, and patients have been changed. I have tried, however, to paint an accurate picture of the patients, family members, and hospital staffs' emotional responses to these seemingly unexplained random happenings. With this in mind, I realize that words cannot ever adequately convey the agony of their pain.

Linda's Story

As Linda entered through the great double doors fronting the hospital where she had worked as an intensive care nurse for six years, she was proud of its outstanding reputation for excellent medical management and surgical expertise. Though she had given up her job as a nurse four years earlier, the hospital complex was still as familiar as a second home. She welcomed the sight of the towering ash-white in-patient center flanked on all sides by a primary care center on the 52-acre complex. Providence Memorial Hospital was the largest hospital in the state. The 530-bed hospital served as a regional referral patient care center, and each year admitted more than 24,000 patients.

Linda's step quickened as she breezed by the information desk, down the pedestrian link, to the hallway which would lead her to the primary care center. "Finally," she thought, "I'll get some answers." Linda had been haunted during the past two weeks with the realization that she had acquired some type of allergy that was consuming her personal life. Her symptoms had become so frightening that she thought she was a prisoner in her own home, fearing to go out even to the next-door neighbor. As she took her seat in the waiting room, she reflected on the subtle onset of her problem and on its dramatic progression.

Before Linda had ever met an allergist, she suspected that there was likely a noninfectious basis to her periodic bouts of sneezing, runny nose, and watery eyes. She used to joke to her best friend that her nose could singlehandedly keep the tissue industry in business. While she suspected that she probably had some type of allergy, she felt that because each "attack" seemed to subside in less than an hour, there was no sense in seeing a doctor about it or, as she put it, making a mountain of a molehill.

When Linda was in her mid-twenties, she became accustomed to living with what she presumed to be hay fever each spring and fall. But she was becoming less blasé about some of the other manifestations of what could very well be allergic reactions to substances in her environment. It was then that she began to experience a number of occasions where she itched all over, as if her skin was one large mosquito bite. And several times, she had broken out in hives, raised red splotchy patches all over her upper body that itched unbearably and looked as horrible as they felt. These eruptions would occur unpredictably at inconvenient times, like when she was on a canoe trip on Lake Superior, 10 miles from shore. They would subside on their own timetable over a variable period, usually minutes to hours, but invariably too long for her liking.

In her thirties, Linda's symptoms became still worse. After meeting and marrying the man of her dreams, an anesthesiologist who also worked at Providence Memorial Hospital, Linda quit her job as an intensive care nurse. It was around this same time that she and her new husband Clark began to notice different and somewhat puzzling symptoms. On one occasion, within minutes after making love, Linda's face became very flushed, her eyes began to tear and swell shut, her entire body became covered in hives and she had the frightening sensation of choking. She also noted with alarm that the area surrounding her vagina was intensely itchy, swollen, and red. For a few months after this puzzling and scary experience, Linda found that what began as a fun and fulfilling sexual relationship became a life of relative celibacy.

Eight months later, she started to experience similar symptoms on several other occasions that seemed to occur after eating various foods at different restaurants. During these times, Linda experienced itchiness and rash over her body, with watering and swelling of her eyes and with a recurrence of the choking sensation. As far as she could tell, every successive episode seemed to bring a slight worsening of her symptoms.

Each time she experienced these symptoms, she found it harder and harder to shrug off these experiences, which she fantasized might even be life-threatening. When Linda was 36 years old and celebrating her fourth wedding anniversary with her husband Clark, she encountered the frightening personal experience that finally transformed the molehill into a mountain in her mind.

Linda and Clark had been planning their special evening for weeks. Clark had been able to purchase 14th row seats for the Elvis Costello Concert at the Winchester Music Center, just 20 minutes from their Federal Hill home. After a wonderfully romantic dinner of seafood and pasta accompanied by a bottle of Sauvignon Blanc from Chateau Margaux at one of the city's finest restaurants, the two were ready to enjoy the music of one of their favorite entertainers. As they took their seats in the concert arena, Linda's face became itchy and flushed. Her eyes and then her whole face began to swell. "Oh no," she thought, "not again!" The itchiness and rash spread and soon her whole body was affected. Costello opened his concert just as Linda started to choke, her throat constricting to a greater degree than ever before. When an individual experiences shortness of breath with a drop in blood pressure, these symptoms are often seen in anaphylactic shock. Linda and Clark became increasingly anxious when Linda began to feel as if she couldn't get enough air, and they quickly left the concert.

It took three days for this episode to subside as Linda took diphenhydramine and other over-the-counter "cold" medicines. While Clark was gratified that her symptoms disappeared, he was very upset about their lost evening. He explained to Linda that he was not concerned about missing the concert, but he was quite worried about losing his wife from anaphylactic shock. Unwilling now to allow Linda to downplay the increasing seriousness of her reactions, Clark called Linda's primary care physician and obtained for Linda the earliest available appointment.

Virginia's Story

Virginia and Bob would be the first to admit it. They were destined to meet and fall in love. Virginia was a country girl from the small West Virginia town of Martinsburg. Though she grew up in a family of modest means supported only by the income of her hard-working bricklayer father, her parents gave her the feeling that she could achieve a limitless destiny and accomplish any dream. Because service and caring for their neighbors and others in the community were integral parts of the core values of her family, Virginia's pursuit of a career in nursing at a prestigious hospital in New York City, Woodrow Wilson Hospital, was consistent with her family's expectations.

Bob was proud to be joining the second generation of physicians in his family. After years of study and dedication, he received his medical degree at the prestigious Brown University School of Medicine. Like his father, Bob's heart was set on a career in family practice. When Bob received his acceptance as an intern at the internationally recognized Woodrow Wilson Hospital, his whole family was pleased; they felt he was making an ideal start on the road to establishing his own family medicine practice in New York City.

Bob worked long hours caring for patients during an internship that was both physically and emotionally demanding. He relied on the support of his colleagues and friends to lift the burden with occasional windows of laughter and conversation. He also appreciated the gentle guidance and assistance of the attractive West Virginia nurse, Virginia, whom he met during the first week of his internship. As they worked together caring for patients, he noted that Virginia had more clinical experience than he did and was able to contribute her insight in ways that often changed patient care. Bob and Virginia's common work ethic and mutual professional respect blossomed into a romance that soon led to marriage.

They decided to set up practice and live in Greenwich Village. This neighborhood was filled with writers, teachers, entertainers, and artists who became their friends and extended family. As Bob's family medicine practice grew in this rich intellectual environment, all of the couple's dreams appeared to be coming true. They were soon blessed by the births of two healthy, handsome boys who were immediately welcomed by their loving, creative extended family. But this utopic period in their lives was shattered suddenly by an unexpected catastrophe that evolved into a four-year nightmare.

One Wednesday afternoon in October, their seemingly idyllic existence was transformed into lives filled with fearful expectations. After returning from work, Virginia mentioned to her husband that she was feeling quite ill. She described experiencing a sudden onset of constant abdominal pain in the lower right portion of her abdomen. This pain, occurring two days before she expected her period, wasn't crampy in nature, but was constant in intensity and caused her to rest motionless on the couch. As Bob comforted her with reassurances, he quickly examined her abdomen by gently placing his hand on her right lower abdominal wall, which elicited exquisite tenderness. Concerned about Virginia's condition, Bob called her gynecologist and primary care physician, Dr. Tim Jones, and asked him to meet them in the Emergency Department of Woodrow Wilson Hospital.

Twenty minutes later in the Emergency Department, Dr. Jones' examination confirmed Bob's description of Virginia's signs and symptoms. He gently pressed his hands on and around each of the organs in her abdomen to discern the nature of the problem, and identified an exquisitely tender tumor-like mass near her uterus. When Dr. Jones pressed down on the right lower portion of her abdomen, Virginia complained of considerable pain that was worsened when he released his hand from her abdomen. He recognized this finding of rebound tenderness, which is a classic symptom that warned of possible peritonitis, a condition caused by irritation and inflammation of the lining of the abdominal cavity.

Dr. Jones made a mental list of the possible causes of her pain. One possible cause was a ruptured ovarian cyst with the spillage of blood into her abdomen and a resultant severe irritation of the lining of her abdominal cavity. Another serious consideration was appendicitis with a ruptured appendix, a situation that releases feces to float freely in the abdominal cavity. As

Dr. Jones discussed these possibilities with Bob and Virginia, Bob tightened his grip on Virginia's hand, realizing that his wife would soon be taken to the operating room. Virginia clearly required surgery. Bob's anxiety was enhanced as he watched the attendants help his beloved wife onto a stretcher that would soon wheel her away to the operating room.

Three hours later Dr. Jones returned from the operating room smiling, and told Bob that Virginia had a ruptured ovarian cyst and that he fully expected her to have a speedy recovery. Hearing this promising news, Bob called his anxious children and then rushed to the recovery room to support his wife. When she returned home four days later, Bob and Virginia were prepared to resume the blissful life that they had created in their Greenwhich Village brownstone. Virginia recovered from her surgery quickly; she was back on her feet both in the home and the office within 10 days of her discharge from the hospital. She still had some lingering discomfort, but it did not interfere with her dual roles as mother and nurse.

Twelve months later, Virginia faced a new agonizing predicament, a uniquely different type of abdominal pain. Though she could not exactly localize the region accounting for the source of her pain, the periodic bouts of cramping nearly brought her to her knees and were accompanied by nausea and vomiting that kept her near the bathroom. When Bob returned home from work, he recognized that his wife's condition was serious, and quickly returned her to the Emergency Department.

Dr. Jones again came to the rescue, finding that Virginia's abdominal condition was dramatically different from the last episode. She now complained of colicky abdominal pain, but could not precisely identify in which region of her abdomen the pain originated. Virginia told the doctor that her pain had begun quite suddenly at quarter past eight o'clock that morning, and that since that time, she couldn't rest or find a comfortable position. She described the miserable nausea that she had been experiencing and the waves of brownish-yellow vomitus. When he put his stethoscope on her abdomen, Dr. Jones heard loud intestinal noises that coincided with the height of Virginia's crampy bouts of pain. He ordered an emergency X-ray examination of her abdomen. When he reviewed the X-ray, he could trace the loops of her small intestine and see that they were distended with gas, confirming his suspicion that Virginia had an acute case of small bowel obstruction.

Intestinal obstruction occurs when the tubelike intestines are blocked and don't allow transport of the intestinal contents. Food and drink, the secretions of the digestive tract, and swallowed air accumulate above the level of the obstruction. Dr. Jones feared an adhesive band at the site of the previous surgical incision caused the obstruction that compressed Virginia's bowel and blocked the passage of intestinal contents. Realizing that patients with intestinal obstruction are best cared for by a general surgeon, he asked Dr. Roland Thomas, Chief of Surgery, to evaluate Virginia's condition.

Dr. Thomas was no stranger to patients with acute intestinal obstruction. During his 20 years of surgical practice, he had encountered numerous patients who developed adhesive bands in their abdominal cavities that caused acute intestinal obstruction. He knew that nasogastric suction would often relieve the intestinal distention and lead to a reopening of the intestinal tract, eliminating the need for surgery. Occasionally, Dr. Thomas' patients would develop another bout of intestinal obstruction, necessitating surgical intervention to divide the adhesive band that compressed the bowel. The surgeon explained to Virginia that she had acute intestinal obstruction; he felt that her condition would respond to nasogastric suction within a 48-hour period. If this conservative treatment did not resolve her intestinal obstruction, Dr. Thomas warned Virginia, surgery would be needed.

In the Emergency Department, Dr. Thomas passed a long, slim nasogastric tube through Virginia's right nostril, down the back of her throat, positioning its end in her stomach. The free end of the nasogastric tube was then attached to a portable electric suction device that continually withdrew swallowed air, digested food, and stomach fluids from Virginia's stomach. This suction was applied in an effort to remove the exerted pressure from the buildup of these substances on her blocked intestines. Dr. Thomas also ordered the placement of an intravenous line (IV) and began fluid replacement therapy to prevent Virginia from becoming dehydrated. Virginia's transfer to the intensive care unit was the beginning of a long 48-hour wait to determine if nasogastric suction had effectively opened her obstructed bowel.

Six hours after nasogastric suction was initiated, Virginia experienced a progressive disappearance of her colicky pain. She had a momentary feeling of euphoria, believing that the disappearance of her abdominal pain was going to be followed by a reopening of her intestinal tract, eliminating the need for surgery. When the nasogastric tube was removed 48 hours later, Virginia's colicky pain recurred. She realized that her dreams of a speedy recovery had vanished, and that surgical exploration would be necessary to reopen her blocked intestine. As Bob sat with his wife before the newest planned surgery, the only circumstance that had changed was that there was a new doctor who would perform the operation. This change in staff gave him a glimmer of hope that Virginia's nightmare would end with a rapid return to her family. Later, Bob found himself again gently brushed aside as the attendant came to take Virginia down the hallway toward the operating room for emergency surgery. Before she left, Bob kissed his wife's heart-shaped face, sending up a small prayer for her safety.

Four hours later, Dr. Thomas returned to the waiting room to tell Bob that the surgery was successfully completed. The operation had revealed thick fibrotic adhesions encasing several loops of Virginia's small intestines, matting them together and accounting for her small bowel obstruction. Dr. Thomas explained that during the surgery, all of the bandlike adhesions were carefully removed, and portions of the adhesions were sent to the Pathology Department for study under a microscope to determine a possible cause for their formation.

Virginia was discharged from the hospital three days later. The pathology report returned, confirming that the tissue sample was a fibrotic adhesion but provided no insight into the underlying cause of the adhesion. Dr. Thomas explained that adhesions form as part of the healing process that goes awry, and are not uncommon after abdominal surgical procedures. His explanation disturbed Virginia, and she asked him, "If adhesions are a natural part of the healing process, does this mean that your surgery may result in another bout of intestinal obstruction?" Dr. Thomas' answer was very disappointing. He explained that there was a small group of patients who experience recurrent episodes of intestinal obstruction after each operation and that the cause for this recurrence was not yet known. He reassured her by saying that patients with recurrent intestinal obstructions are rarely encountered. In fact, he had only had twenty such patients in his extensive operative experience.

One year after the operation for bowel obstruction and two years after her initial surgery to repair the ruptured ovarian cyst, Virginia again found herself in the Emergency Department of Woodrow Wilson Hospital. Exhausted by a sleepless night, she had spent the previous eleven hours vomiting and writhing with crampy pain that was achingly reminiscent of her previous episode of acute intestinal obstruction. Dr. Thomas was awakened by the 5 A.M. call that informed him that Virginia urgently needed care. He hurried to the Emergency Department to meet Virginia and Bob. The history she gave of her illness and her physical examination convinced Dr. Thomas that Virginia was suffering from a recurrence of intestinal obstruction. Her abdominal X-ray confirmed his suspicion. His treatment came as no surprise to Virginia; a nasogastric tube, intravenous fluids, and a gentle reminder that surgery might be necessary to relieve the obstruction if the colicky pain persisted after an attempt to decompress her bowel with nasogastric suction. Virginia was watched carefully for her anticipated disappearance of the obstruction, which persisted after the 48-hour observation period. Virginia was soon to learn that she was one of a select group of individuals who experienced recurrent acute intestinal obstruction after surgery, a condition for which there is no answer. For the third time, Virginia was taken for emergency surgery.

When he reexplored her abdomen, Dr. Thomas again found a conglomeration of filmy and fibrotic adhesive bands connecting the coils of Virginia's intestines. He scowled briefly behind his mask, and then quickly set to the task of releasing the adhesive bands while taking extreme care to avoid injuring the tissues. Before closing the abdominal incision, he collected another sample of the cut adhesions to send to the pathologist, in hopes of finding an answer to her challenging illness. The pathologist's report was erudite and eloquent, but offered no insight into the cause of the adhesions.

At her follow-up appointment, Virginia appeared to be healing without incident but seemed particularly withdrawn. When pressed, she mentioned that her relationship with Bob had been strained. Bob had temporarily hired a replacement nurse for the office, and Virginia felt somewhat displaced. She also complained of feeling depressed about the "ugly" pink scar on her belly that was tender and made her feel unattractive. But Virginia was perhaps most concerned with the effect these recurrent surgical problems had on her eldest son, who now refused to leave the house after returning from school each day, scared that his mother would need him. Virginia was anxious to see an end to this ordeal, and looked forward to a long stretch of time without the need for medical care.

One evening, roughly three months after Virginia was discharged from the hospital, Bob returned home to find his wife sobbing. She begged him to hold her, but wouldn't tell Bob what was wrong. Her clammy skin spoke of her recurring nightmare, and when she broke away from his embrace, Bob could see a mixture of pain and fear on Virginia's face. She told Bob that all day she had been tormented by the cramping pain and vomiting that she feared signaled that her bowels were again obstructed. Virginia's anguish intensified as she cried out that she could not bear the thought of another possible surgery. Cognizant of her urgent need of medical care, Bob assisted his weakened wife into their sedan.

Two days later, Bob found himself wandering the hospital cafeteria, gazing idly at the food displays without any intention of eating. He needed a distraction from worrying about his wife, who was once again in the operating room. Dr. Thomas' surgical skill was never in doubt. Rather, Bob could not help but return again and again in his mind to the sight of Virginia's tears over the thought of another operation. And this time, only three months had elapsed. Was her situation getting still worse? Would they ever be free of this recurring torment?

Dr. Thomas, too, was frustrated and concerned. In the operation, Virginia's small intestines again demonstrated a twisting network of fibrotic adhesions. Dr. Thomas was exasperated by his inability to provide Virginia with the ultimate comfort of knowing that they could prevent a repeat episode of this painful and dangerous condition. For this, he would need to know the cause for her excessive adhesion formation. In his continued search for a solution to Virginia's recurrent illness, Dr. Thomas resolved to send the biopsy of the adhesions to another major regional medical center to see if they could determine the cause. They had to find a way to stop this cycle of intolerable pain and suffering that was turning a confident and proud West Virginia woman into a sad, despondent and fearful little girl.

Peter's Story

When Peter entered the office of his Honolulu architectural firm that morning, his secretary, Sandy, noted that he was visibly disturbed. And not just a little. Peter's grimace, combined with his unusually large size, contributed to a formidable picture. Without stopping for his customarily warm greeting and cup of coffee, Peter ducked into the office with little to say except to request that Sandy get his physician on the line. She quickly consulted the Rolodex and dialed the doctor's office, waiting to hear Dr. Deborah Campbell's voice before she patched through the call.

Peter sat behind the tall Koa wood desk and took in the vista outside his window. He gazed out across Honolulu harbor, his eyes finding walls of ominous dark gray clouds loaded with rain spanning the horizon. Slowly his vision shifted back to the familiar and friendly sight of the docks along the edge of the harbor.

A distant car horn broke Peter's concentration and brought him back to the reorganization of his day, and the imminent call from his doctor. Dr. Campbell was always available for his calls, and had a reputation throughout the islands for competence, compassion and great attention for detail.

Despite a good relationship with his internist, Peter was tired of doctors and of the recent bout of health problems that had materialized in the preceding months. Having just turned 45 years of age, he still thought of himself as young and athletic, and considered that he should be as free of physical concerns as he had been during the preceding 44 years. Several months earlier he had noticed a slight bulge that seemed to appear suddenly in his lower right abdomen. It was tender at times, and noticeably increased in tenderness when he coughed. Constipation had been a challenging problem for him throughout his life, requiring the frequent use of laxatives. Now Peter started to notice that if he had to strain when using the bathroom, the area near the bulge would ache.

At first Peter downplayed the importance of the pain and the bulge in his lower right abdomen, but when he saw blood on the surface of his stool one morning, his denial of his illness disappeared. He quickly sought medical help. A visit to Dr. Campbell's office revealed that he had a hernia. She explained that his condition was most likely a direct inguinal (groin) hernia, and explained that the bulge was caused by the protrusion of Peter's intestines through an area of his abdominal wall that had been weakened by repeated episodes of straining during defecation. She emphasized that it was important that the hernia be repaired with surgery to prevent his intestines from being trapped in the hernial sac, which could result in dire consequences.

Dr. Campbell was also concerned that her examination confirmed the presence of blood in Peter's stool. She commented that prior to any surgical repair of his hernia, Peter would require a further test, an air-contrast barium enema, to rule out the possibility of colon cancer. Peter tried to maintain his impassive appearance as he felt Dr. Campbell's words strike fear into his heart. Initially quite anxious to hear that he would need surgery to correct the problem, the word "cancer" pierced him like a burning spear and its effect continued to smolder in his tight chest. His mother had died of colon cancer, and his grandfather of lung cancer. He was speechless in his apprehension and he had difficulty following the rest of Dr. Campbell's instructions. The word "cancer" resonated through his mind as he impatiently waited for the diagnostic test.

Appreciating his distress, his doctor made an early appointment for him to have the diagnostic procedure the following morning. She told Peter that he should not eat or drink anything except clear liquids for the rest of the day, and gave him a five liter-sized bottle of a clear solution called GoLYTELY that he had to finish during the rest of that day. He was to return home after leaving her office and be certain to drink all five liters in order to get his bowels ready for the barium X-ray. She explained that the liquid was a cathartic that would help to empty his intestines, and that he would need to be in close proximity to his bathroom.

The barium examination showed no evidence of cancer. Though he felt emotionally drained during the three days after the X-ray and before he could get the definitive word from the radiologist, all Peter would recall was his relief that the X-ray results were normal. He was so comforted by Dr. Campbell's good news that he actually viewed the surgical correction of his hernia as an opportunity to resume his busy personal and professional life without the discomfort of the bulge in his lower abdominal wall.

Dr. Campbell met with Peter again to discuss exactly what he could expect on the day of his surgery. She referred him to a respected and talented surgeon, Dr. Richard Smith, with whom she had had a long professional relationship, and promised to check in on him the day that he was admitted to the hospital. The operation to repair his hernia was performed under local anesthesia and took only 90 minutes. Dr. Smith's speed was considered by many to be testimony for his surgical excellence. Peter was able to return to work 10 days after his surgery and was instructed to avoid heavy lifting. Apart from some mild discomfort around his healing incision, Peter felt well and received good reports during his postoperative appointment with his surgeon.

Now six weeks out from his surgery, Peter's worried eyes stared vacantly at the timeless beauty of Honolulu harbor bordered by the new shops and restaurants that formed Honolulu's popular Restaurant Row. During the last two weeks, things had not gone so well for Peter. He began to notice increasing discomfort in that same right lower abdominal region. While lying in bed that morning, he had gingerly explored the area, and had found a hard lump about two and one-half inches in diameter that laid beneath the site of his surgical incision. Somewhat bewildered at first, he was suddenly startled by the thought that the hard lump could be cancer. Peter began to wonder about the accuracy of the barium X-ray procedure. "Was this a new cancer?" he thought. "Or was this evidence of spread of a cancer from his bowel undetected during the X-ray examination." Peter tried to swallow his fearful thoughts as he awaited Dr. Campbell's call. He anxiously sat by the phone, hoping to hear Dr. Campbell's voice that would have a less frightening explanation for this unexplained mass than his supposition of a cancer that was spreading through his body.

Jack and Renee's Story

In the examination room in the infertility clinic at the prestigious Western Virginia Medical School, Renee was about to be examined for what seemed like the hundredth time in the last five years. Lying on the narrow, sterile examination table, Renee's short frame was enveloped by the crackling paper sheaths and white linens that provided for her modesty. Hearing his sigh, Renee turned to glance at her carrot-topped husband Jack, sitting two feet away on one of the three straight-backed plastic chairs that lined the wall of the room.

Jack and Renee, now 39 and 37 respectively, first met in their early twenties when Renee was a recent college graduate with visions of a successful career in TV journalism. Jack was a news writer, and Renee, an ambitious field reporter, for the local NBC news affiliate in Los Angeles. Thrown together on the job, the two found they shared a unique camaraderie on assignment, and their affection for each other grew.

The couple married the year that Renee turned 30, and Jack and Renee's honeymoon lasted well into the second year of their marriage. They managed to save some money and put it aside to buy a house. After another year, Renee's proverbial biologic clock stopped ticking and started booming. Her urge to have children was so strong that she started looking at other people's children with thoughts like, "Ooh! I'd take that one." She would fawn over the toddlers in the shore break when she and Jack spent their weekends at the beach, and peer into each baby carriage that rolled within a half block radius of any given path she took.

Jack's emotions did not at first match her overwhelming enthusiasm to procreate. He was in the midst of finalizing his preparations to return to school, and had cast out applications for graduate school in a wide net that spanned the major universities and colleges of the East and West Coasts of the United States. When Jack accepted a position at the Western Virginia Law School, Renee secretly rejoiced at leaving the hustle of her lucrative journalism career, thinking that the absence of stress of the news business would contribute positively toward starting a new family and that Charlotte, Virginia, would be an ideal setting for child-rearing compared with the urban tensions and excitements of Los Angeles.

Jack and Renee packed a U-Haul and their two cars and were settled in a two-story colonial rental on a quiet, tree-lined street within four weeks of their arrival in Charlotte. After her initial three months of difficulty finding a suitable job in a college town flooded with a well-educated work force, Renee circulated fliers and established a new career doing free-lance ghost writing and editorial work.

A little over a year after Jack started law school, he arrived home one day with a dozen pink roses and asked, almost shyly, if she was ready to start a family. It was a climactic and memorable moment for them both as they watched the birth control pills sail into the trash, pills that the couple had faithfully remembered for many years.

Months went by, and Renee didn't conceive. At first, she was unconcerned that she was not getting pregnant. Renee assumed that, because of her age, it might take her longer to become pregnant than it would take her friends in their early twenties. But after two years of passionate sexual encounters with her husband, the only outcome was the repetition of her menstrual cycle. With renewed enthusiasm, Renee made an appointment to see a gynecologist, Dr. David Blake, who was an infertility specialist recognized throughout the world.

The soothing decor of Dr. Blake's office complemented the physician's bedside manner. After a long discussion and a thorough physical exam, Dr. Blake suggested Renee dress and join him in his office. There he explained that Renee would need to take her daily temperature, a basal body temperature reading taken each morning after awakening but before she rose from bed. They arranged for a follow-up appointment, and the next month Renee returned faithfully with her temperature chart in hand and her husband Jack by her side. As the three sat separated by a desk cluttered with journals and files, Dr. Blake enumerated additional recommendations.

Dr. Blake, Renee, and Jack constructed a careful schedule in which the doctor advised intercourse every two days around the time Renee ovulated. They left Dr. Blake's office with their minds spinning full of detailed instructions, but with renewed hope and buoyed spirits. Despite the scheduled sex, Jack still always seemed in the mood. They did not allow the regimentation of their sex life to disturb them, but instead approached sex enthusiastically, each time considering that, "This could be the time." But every month, Renee's periods appeared with frustrating regularity, every 28 to 32 days.

One year later, on a return visit to Dr. Blake's office, he suggested that they try another approach. He recommended that they obtain a hysterosalpingogram, an X-ray examination of Renee's uterus and fallopian tubes that could reveal any blockages or abnormalities. He explained that during the test a special dye would be injected into her fallopian tubes while sequential X-rays were taken. Renee was more than willing to undergo any procedure that could help target a specific problem in her ability to get pregnant. The hysterosalpingogram revealed a left-sided tubal blockage. Dr. Blake explained to

Renee and Jake that tubal blockage was a common cause of female infertility; however, these blockages are usually bilateral. Because Renee's tubular blockage was only on the left, he did not feel that this was the sole cause of her infertility. Not wanting to subject Renee to an unnecessary surgery to correct this unilateral blockage, Dr. Blake put Renee on Clomid (clomiphene citrate), which he described as a drug that encourages ovulation, and that, as a side effect, might result in a multiple birth, most often twins. Renee expressed eagerness to take the medication and felt that the possibility that she could have twins would be viewed as a double blessing. Renee took the drug for five days each month. Other than experiencing startling hot flashes, she had little difficulty with the medication. Dr. Blake tracked her progress each month, and slowly increased Renee's dosage over the next three months from 50 mg to 100 mg each day. Each month Renee thought, "Well this month, it will work." But their continuing lack of success brought Renee to despair.

Meanwhile, a fall from his 10-speed bike left Jack with a torn shoulder and made him a less willing participant in his and Renee's scheduled sexual encounters. His invitation to join a prestigious law firm provided a brief celebration for the couple and an occasion for a two-week vacation to the Virgin Islands.

The couple returned safely to their Charlotte home and began unpacking, readying themselves for the return to the chaos of the real world. Jack asked Renee if she would enjoy having a small supper before bedtime. Renee considered this option and was puzzled that she had little or no appetite. She encouraged Jack to enjoy supper while she would continue to unpack his shaving kit and her toiletries. The vacation ended as it began, with Renee encircled in Jack's loving arms as they fell asleep in bed. Three hours later, at 3:00 A.M. Renee was awakened by a pain in her abdomen. Her constant pain seemed to be localized around her belly button and was associated with a continued disinterest in eating. Initially, she thought it might have been some of the food that she ate during her recent plane flight, no cause for concern. The pain, however, grew worse, and Renee became nauseated. She awoke Jack and asked for his assistance, as she walked into the bathroom, anticipating that she might vomit. As she sat on a chair near the sink, Renee updated Jack on the progression of her symptoms. Her pain had migrated now to the right lower portion of her abdominal wall. As she applied direct pressure to the skin overlying this area, the pain worsened, being relieved by removing her hand from her abdominal wall. Terrified over what could be happening to his wife, Jack immediately dialed 9-1-1. He ran back to the bathroom where he held his wife tightly, comforting her as best he could until the paramedics arrived.

In the Emergency Department, Renee was quickly and thoroughly examined by the emergency physician, Dr. Mary Smith. Renee had a low-grade fever (37.9° C). When placing a stethoscope on her abdomen, the doctor heard diminished bowel sounds. As the doctor pressed on the lower right side of her abdomen, Renee cried out in pain and when she lifted his hand off of her abdomen, she almost jumped off of the table, the pain was so intense. A pelvic exam was performed which elicited pain in the same area; her rectal exam was normal. Knowing that Renee's history and clinical presentation were consistent with acute appendicitis, Dr. Smith immediately notified Dr. Walter Boyd, the surgeon on call to evaluate Renee for a possible emergency appendectomy. Anticipating that Dr. Boyd would agree with her clinical diagnosis, she started the administration of intravenous fluids containing antibiotics that reduce the incidence of postoperative infection. Renee clung to Jack's hand as she impatiently awaited the arrival of Dr. Boyd. She also insisted that Dr. Blake be notified because he had been working so closely with the couple for years. She valued his opinion more than any other person.

It was fortuitous that Dr. Blake was in the hospital seeing another patient when he learned about Renee's call for help. So he and Dr. Boyd arrived almost simultaneously to Renee's room in the Emergency Department. Following further examination, both doctors readily agreed with the astute emergency physician's diagnosis of acute appendicitis. Dr. Boyd explained to Renee and Jack that Renee's pain was most likely secondary to an inflammation of the appendix. Renee was so terrified of surgery that she almost refused; however, the pain was too much to bear. She consented to the surgery. Jack, who had never seen his wife so sick and weak, was overwhelmed by the fear of losing her. Reluctantly he released her hand as she was wheeled away on a gurney in preparation for surgery. Dr. Blake escorted Jack to the waiting room where he assuaged some of Jack's fears. Jack, unable to relax, paced the waiting room for the next two hours as he expectantly awaited Dr. Boyd's confirmation that surgery was successful.

Jack received this good news as Dr. Boyd entered the waiting room dressed in surgical scrubs with a large grin on his face. "Everything is fine, Jack. We made a three-inch-long incision in your wife's right lower abdominal wall, right over the area where her appendix lies. I found exactly what I expected—an inflamed appendix. It was not perforated. I removed it without difficulty. Renee is in the intensive care unit. She's doing well, but still a little groggy from the anesthesia. She's asking for you." Jack thanked Dr. Boyd, breathed a sigh of relief, and raced to his wife's side. He stayed by her side throughout her short hospital stay. Renee was a healthy woman who healed quickly and was ready to return home with her husband two days later. As her memories of her serious illness slowly disappeared, Renee began to refocus on what appeared to be the most important goal of her life. She diligently continued her clomiphene and followed all of the instructions that Dr. Blake had enumerated and the two resumed love-making with a new intense passion. To no avail, Renee continued to have her periods returning to the dreaded 30-day menstrual cycle.

Three months after her life-threatening appendectomy, Renee received a surprising call from Dr. Blake, asking that she and her husband return to his office. An unplanned personal telephone call from her physician was a surprise to her because she had never previously had a physician instigate an impromptu call. Her mind began to wander over the possible reasons for Dr. Blake's call. She doubted seriously if the intention of this call was to give her good news, but rather one of sharing bad news in a setting where she would be supported by her beloved husband. By the time of her appointment, she was almost hysterical, anticipating that Dr. Blake would be announcing the finding of a serious life-threatening condition or even the worst possibility—announcing that she was infertile and could not conceive a child. Dr. Blake had so captivated their attention that they memorized his every word. "Renee, I want to emphasize to you the importance of the appendectomy that removed your inflamed appendix before it perforated. This emergency operative procedure saved your life. While you are making a remarkable physical recovery, I am worried that this abdominal infectious process, appendicitis, may have caused the development of thin bands or strings that cover the opening of your other fallopian tube." Consequently he recommended a repeat hysterosalpingogram to identify the presence of blockage of her right fallopian tube secondary to these adhesions. Renee readily agreed to the X-ray. Dr. Blake's prediction of the development of blockage of her right fallopian tube was confirmed by the X-ray. What was previously a unilateral left-sided tubal blockage was now a bilateral tubal blockage. With a look of enormous despair and disappointment, Renee asked Dr. Blake for a sign of hope. "Is there any medication or surgical procedure that will open the blockage of my tubes so that I can have my baby?" As he responded, Dr. Blake had an air of confidence and optimism that filled the room with hope.

Dr. Blake explained to Renee that the next course of action would be a new surgical procedure. This procedure involved a combination of new microsurgical techniques with the use of small endoscopes. The endoscopes were narrow fiberoptic tubes through which the obstetrician would be able to visualize the reproductive system. When the blockage was identified, it could be reopened using delicate fine microsurgical instruments. A biopsy of the tissue covering the openings of the tubes would be obtained to facilitate understanding of the cause of infertility.

Having recently successfully undergone the emergency appendectomy, Renee was almost optimistic at the prospects of the planned surgery. She would do anything to uncover this mystery. When she explained the situation to Jack, he was not as eager for Renee to have surgery. He loved Renee, pregnant or not, and did not think she needed to be taking so many risks. Sensing Renee's renewed hope and the excitement it brought her, Jack could not bring himself to talk her out of the operation. Dr. Blake scheduled Renee for a laparoscopy and reconstructive microsurgery. The laparoscopic procedure involved the insertion of a fiberoptic scope in a small incision near Renee's navel. The image was transmitted to a television monitor and allowed Dr. Blake to examine her uterus, ovaries, fallopian tubes, and other abdominal structures without having to make a large abdominal incision. This laparoscopic procedure revealed extensive adhesions that formed a web around Renee's ovaries and swollen fallopian tubes.

He performed a procedure known as a microsurgical tuboplasty that repaired Renee's blocked fallopian tubes and removed the adhesions around her ovaries. Dr. Blake collected samples of tissue from the adhesions and sent them to pathology for interpretation. He hoped this would solve the puzzle of the new adhesion formation.

Dr. Blake scheduled a postoperative appointment in his office one week later to discuss the results of the pathology report. Renee counted the days until she could find out exactly what was keeping her from having a baby. What was forming these awful adhesions that were robbing her of her womanhood? She hoped that with these answers would come a solution. Time seemed to stand still as the waiting game continued for Renee and Jack.

Jim's Story

Jim didn't sing in the choir any more; he hadn't for over three months. Still wooed by all three Protestant churches in the small southern Ohio town, the 73-year-old white-haired tenor had to take a break when his eyesight prohibited him from making out the tiny text on the musical scores. The First Methodist choir director called him periodically to beg his return, and Jim, too, was anxious to rejoin the choir; singing remained one of the highlights of his retired life.

Jim and his wife Mary had made Glenville, Ohio, their home for over 50 years. In the early days, Jim landed a job as a sheet metal worker for the C&O railroad. Years of loyal hard work resulted in promotions that allowed him to retire as a foreman with a generous railroad pension. Jim met Mary when she was an elementary school teacher at Kingsbury Elementary on Vernon Street, near the center of town. Before the birth of their three daughters, Mary taught third grade in the old-fashioned red brick two-story building with its hardwood floors and slate blackboards. She and Jim still reminisced about the bell tower that once rang to signal the start of each school day. The bell tower had been torn down in the 1960's to accommodate renovations to the school, long after Mary left her teaching position to concentrate her efforts in their home.

Their big green house on South Sixth Street that had been home for so long was now relatively empty. Their daughters, one in Cincinnati, one in Cleveland, and one nearby in Glenville, had grown children of their own. Mary spent her summers in the garden and her winters knitting. Jim had been an avid Cincinnati Reds and Cincinnati Bengals fan longer than anyone remembered. When he wasn't watching sports, he was reading the local newspaper, *The Glenville Tribune*. At least, that was true before the recent trouble with his vision.

Over the last year, Jim had noticed increasing difficulty reading and seeing street signs. At first, images seemed a little blurred. With time, however, he noticed that he could see less and less. He was afraid that his vision would soon fail altogether. It was a parking lot fender bender at the grocery store that finally spurred Jim to make an appointment with his family practitioner to look into the problem.

Dr. Paul Green scheduled an appointment for Jim the following week, and incorporated an eye examination into Jim's annual physical. After his physical examination, Dr. Green explained to Jim that there was evidence of cataract formation in both of Jim's eyes. Dr. Green felt that the right eye demonstrated what was probably early cataract formation (because it was not visible to the unaided eye), but the cataract formation in the left eye was advanced, and the bluish white hazy plaque could be seen by anyone who looked.

Using an ophthalmoscope to examine a normal eye, a physician expects to see a red shiny reflection from the region of the pupil, similar in nature to the reflection seen from the eyes of animals caught in headlights by the side of the road. But when Dr. Green examined Jim's left eye with an ophthalmoscope, the red reflex was very poor, suggesting a dense cataract. The partial cataract in the right eye appeared black against the red reflex. Dr. Green left the examination room momentarily, returning with a referral for Jim to see his ophthalmologist. The doctor suggested that the ophthalmologist could best discuss treatment options, but that surgery to remove one or both of the cataracts would probably be a consideration.

Jim's ophthalmologist, Dr. Sarah Fedson, had a busy practice despite her small town location. In part, this was because Jim's condition was so common. Cataract formation is a frequent malady for elders, and Dr. Fedson often reminded her patients that some degree of cataract formation is to be expected in all persons over age 70. In fact, she told patients, age-related cataract formation occurs in 50 percent of individuals between ages 65 and 74, and in about 70 percent of people over age 75. While cataracts account for the most common cause of visual loss in the United

States untreatable with glasses, they are one of the most success-fully treated conditions in all of surgery.

When she examined Jim, Dr. Fedson confirmed that Jim had cataracts in both eyes. She tested his visual acuity, or the limits of his ability to see, using a well-illuminated Snellen chart. With glasses, the visual acuity of his left eye could not be corrected to better than 20/100; with the right eye he could read the 20/80 line with best correction. Dr. Fedson told Jim that this examina-tion indicated moderate low vision in his right eye and severe low vision in his left eye. She elaborated that his present visual acuity would be insufficient for a driver's license; neither eye would pass such a test. The rest of Jim's eye examination demon-strated no other problems. Jim's retina and optic nerve were nor-mal.

Dr. Fedson asked Jim to meet with her in her office. "When does your vision bother you?" was her first question. "Does your eyesight keep you from doing what you need and want to do?" After a brief pause, Jim confided that he had been worried for some time about losing his sight. He shared with Dr. Fedson his fear that he would lose the ability to take his wife, Mary, who had never learned to drive, to her hairdresser, to the gro-cery store, and to her doctor's appointments. Even in the day-time, he now had difficulty seeing traffic signs. Jim also told Dr. Fedson of his inability to read without strong magnifiers, and that even with magnification, his reading speed seemed slowed.

Jim noticed Dr. Fedson's careful attention as he spoke. When she replied to his comments, he was aware that she seemed to choose her words with the same deliberate care with which she listened. "Approximately 1.5 million cataract extractions are per-formed each year in America," Dr. Fedson told Jim. "Although no surgery is without risk, cataract extractions are very simple and successful procedures." She went on to explain that for Jim, she would recommend surgery. "Without surgery, you will not

be able to do these things that you need and want to do," Dr. Fedson said.

Jim knew several friends who had experienced dramatic improvements in vision following cataract surgery. After a short period of consideration, he welcomed the notion of having the procedure. Dr. Fedson explained that she would prefer to correct only the left eye first; they could later address the need for future surgery involving the right eye. During the procedure to remove the lens with the cataract from the lens capsule of the left eye, she would implant a plastic lens.

Dr. Fedson reviewed the possible risks of the procedure. She warned Jim that some patients developed severe reddening of their eyes following cataract surgery from unknown causes. This inflammatory process rarely results in blindness. Jim carefully weighed this potential serious complication against the real consequences of social isolation from his progressive loss of vision. He immediately decided to choose surgery so that he could continue to enjoy seeing the beauties of life. Jim signed the consent form, and together with Dr. Fedson, identified a date for the surgery.

The operation was swift and uncomplicated, and Jim was told that he would be able to return home the same day. His left eye was covered by an antibiotic ointment, a patch, and a metal eye shield. Jim was given many instructions for care; among them he was told not to read, watch television, or leave the house (except for office visits) until Dr. Fedson gave him clearance. Three follow-up appointments were scheduled during each of the first two weeks after the operation. Once home, Mary kept Jim comfortable, providing pillows to help keep his head erect while he dozed in his favorite chair, and reading to him from *The Glenville Tribune* and *Reader's Digest* to help pass the time.

At his first postoperative check, Dr. Fedson removed the metal shield and eye patch. She was dismayed by what she saw. Jim had returned with severe inflammation of the iris of his eye.

The iris, the thin colored sheet of tissue that surrounds the pupil and gives the eye its characteristic blue, green, or brown appearance, lies in front of the lens. It responds to inflammation by becomming flushed, engorged with blood, and by narrowing the pupil opening to a pinpoint. The inflammation also caused Jim's left eye to look cloudy, and Dr. Fedson could see a layered level of pus in the eye's foremost chamber, like a half-filled glass of milk. She noted in Jim's chart the diagnosis of early endophthalmitis (inflammation of the eye) characterized by early hypopyon formation (pus level) and anterior vitreous cellularity (cloudiness in the foremost chamber of the eye). Because bacteria and irritant substances can both cause this type of reaction, Dr. Fedson decided to insert a needle into Jim's eye to withdraw a sample of the pus. Analysis of the inflammatory fluid would allow her to determine the cause of the inflammation, and thereby ensure appropriate treatment. The needle tap would be a risky procedure and the eye could, in fact, be lost if there were complications, but it was critical to determine what was causing the inflammatory reaction in Jim's eye.

Jim was shocked by the development of this operative complication. Sight in his left eye was his expectation, rather than blindness. He also realized that the risk for the diagnosis for the inflammation exceeded that for the cataract surgery. Regardless of the outcome of this diagnostic test, he silently resolved, "I'll never let her touch my right eye."

———

Our modern hospitals are marked by towering buildings that have a self-contained, carefully controlled environment. These contemporary healthcare centers are designed to be ideal places to work, tailored to human comfort. Patients treated in these facilities have the expectation that they will receive the physical and emotional support that is needed to care effectively for their illness. The dedicated hospital personnel take special precautions to prevent transmission of the patient's illnesses.

With the building regulation codes, neither the patients nor the hospital personnel would believe that the hospital environment could make them ill.

Because hospitals have this loving, protective aura, most patients anticipate that their treatments will have favorable outcomes. When the patient's hospital course is interrupted by a worsening of his condition, a patient may even take full responsibility for this misfortune. Because he attributes his misfortunes to presumably unavoidable causes, he may even assume the persona of being a "loser" who is destined to have bad luck. When the patient accepts this heavy responsibility, that patient's ill-fated complication appears to be an unexplained random happening.

CHAPTER TWO

The Mote That Binds

"It must be heartening to undergraduate medical students to see how fallible their professors are. It must be even more reassuring to them to hear their teachers confess their errors, pointing out how, at various stages in the illness, a more astute and sensitive appraisal of the situation might have had a better and happier ending."

Dr. Owen H. Wangensteen

All the seemingly unrelated events in the preceding chapter have their basis in a single, well-defined factor that elicits an abnormal and exaggerated disease process in the patient. In this chapter we explore that single, well-defined factor. We begin with Linda's story.

Linda's Story

Sitting in the large blue waiting area with a three-month-old copy of *Time* magazine unopened on her lap, Linda was anxious for the word that her family physician, Dr. Christopher Cooper, was ready to see her. Linda's eyes had begun to water two minutes after she arrived, and five soaked tissues lined the plastic seat to her left, remnants of a sneezing attack that brought a mixture of kind blessings and disgusted grimaces from the other waiting patients seated nearby.

Linda's appointment was short. After asking Linda questions and performing a physical examination focused on the assessment of her skin, respiratory system, and major organ systems, Dr. Cooper referred Linda to an allergy specialist. Dr. Dunn belonged to a group practice specializing in allergy and immunology. The four physicians shared a bright, modernly furnished office filled with sunlight and beautiful artificial tropical plants selected so they would brighten the office without presenting allergens to the unsuspecting patient. Linda liked the airy feel of the waiting room with its pine hardwood floor and vaulted ceiling, and quickly discovered that she also rather liked Dr. Dunn. He and Linda quickly established a rapport as they reviewed her history of symptoms: her long-time experience with itchy skin, intermittent hives, hay fever, and the recent episodes involving choking sensations and difficulty breathing.

Upon examination, Dr. Dunn's initial impression was that Linda was a strong, athletic woman, as confirmed by her rather slim, muscular physique, a manifestation of her regular aerobic conditioning program. The appearance of her skin contrasted dramatically with the underlying healthy, muscular tissue. He noted that the skin of her face had a reddened, bumpy rash that had a cobblestone-like appearance. Linda also had several patches of eczema on her neck and lower abdomen that appeared as a dark, thick, dry, scaly rash. The once-white part of her eyes that surrounded her dark blue irises now were reddened and filled with moisture, giving the mistaken impression that she was on the verge of tears. On Dr. Dunn's close examination, this reddened portion of her eyes had a grainy appearance. Her nasal airways were full of a clear discharge and were partially blocked by the swollen, reddened membranes lining her nasal canals. When he placed his stethoscope on Linda's chest, Dr. Dunn could detect a high-pitched wheezing sound as she exhaled. The wheeze indicated a narrowing of the airways in her lungs due to inflammation, a finding consistent with his impression that Linda had a mild case of early asthma that was not severe enough to interfere with her physical endurance. Convinced that Linda was having a severe allergic reaction that was beginning to affect her entire body, Dr. Dunn began the long search for the allergen that was the culprit for her potentially life-threatening allergic responses.

Linda's blood tests for red and white blood cells and for serum electrolytes demonstrated normal counts and concentrations. Allergy skin testing revealed a strongly positive reaction to several pollens (trees, ragweed, and other weeds), house dust, mold, and to a few foods: spinach and potato.

On the basis of the results of skin testing, Dr. Dunn told Linda that his initial clinical impression was that Linda's severe allergic responses were caused by food-induced allergic reactions, possibly to spinach, potato, or even wine. Linda was instructed to keep a food diary and avoid eating potatoes and spinach. Dr. Dunn was also concerned about Linda's reports of swelling and itching around her vagina after sexual contact with Clark. He suspected that she may be allergic to one of the components in her husband's ejaculate. The allergist strongly recommended sexual abstinence, but he told Linda that the use of a latex condom would be permitted until they performed further skin and blood tests to clarify the problem. Before she left the hospital, Dr. Dunn provided Linda with an emergency epinephrine kit, like that used by persons allergic to bee venom. He told her to keep the kit with her at all times and showed her how to inject herself with epinephrine in the event that she experienced another severe reaction that limited her ability to breathe.

Dr. Dunn's thorough physical examination as well as his apparently successful search were comforting to Linda; however, Dr. Dunn was careful to warn Linda that she must have realistic expectations in the event that he had not identified the true culprit for her severe allergic reactions. He assured her that, even if this search was a long journey, he believed that he would find the allergen as well as a solution to the problem.

When Linda returned home that evening, she recounted each detail of her emotionally exhausting day to her husband. Clark was surprised by the variety of plant allergies that Linda had acquired, somewhat taken aback by the newly diagnosed food allergies, and especially shocked by the suggestion that Linda may be allergic to his seminal fluid. Clark agreed to attend a luncheon appointment with Dr. Dunn the following week, anxious to disprove this hypothesis. His concerns about their sexual intimacy were overshadowed by his fears of a fatal allergic reaction. As he remembered his wife's almost fatal episode of anaphylactic shock, Clark vowed to avoid any sexual relations with Linda until the issue was resolved.

The following day at the dentist's office, Linda had her first terrifying opportunity to use the Epi-pen in the epinephrine injection kit that Dr. Dunn gave her. As the dental hygienist cleaned her teeth, Linda experienced the onset of a severe allergic reaction. Hives covered her face and the lining of her mouth swelled upon contact with the rubber dental dam. The hives were followed by generalized swelling of her face and an itchy feeling of her skin that began to spread throughout her body. Her heart began to beat much faster than normal, and she experienced profound shortness of breath. She could even hear the wheezing of air as she tried to exhale. Linda remained motionless, paralyzed by the fear that she was going to die.

Fortunately, Linda's dentist came to the rescue. When the dentist saw the Epi-pen in her open purse, he immediately administered the life-saving epinephrine injection while his hygienist called the paramedics. Linda was taken to the emergency department at Providence Memorial Hospital where she was given supplemental oxygen while her blood oxygen was continuously monitored. Linda received one repeat dose of epinephrine and a potent antihistamine medication. She was watched carefully to ensure that her condition did not deteriorate. Clark was summoned to the emergency department from his on-call room in anesthesiology. His arrival in the Emergency Department brought the first sense of calm to Linda during the ordeal. When all signs of her allergic reaction disappeared, four hours after her arrival in the Emergency

Department, she was discharged with a new Epi-pen and anti-histamine medications.

When Clark and Linda returned to the allergist's office, Dr. Dunn questioned her in detail about this most recent episode of anaphylactic shock. Linda associated the allergic reaction with the placement of the rubber dental dam in her mouth. Intrigued by the agent that supposedly precipitated the allergic reaction, Dr. Dunn pursued further questioning about her exposure to natural latex rubber products. Even though he had known of Linda's previous career as an intensive care nurse who repeatedly wore latex gloves, he had not thought of her as an individual at high risk for latex allergy. Her positive skin test reactions to food made him believe that the foods were the causal factors of her allergic reactions. Because he had recently read scientific reports that demonstrated a unique cross-reactivity between natural rubber latex and foods, he now realized that she could be allergic to the natural rubber latex as well as certain unique foods.

As Dr. Dunn incriminated natural rubber latex as the causal factor of her allergic reactions, the mystery of her illness seemed closer to being solved. Her suspected allergic reaction to her husband's semen after sexual intercourse could, in actuality, be related to their frequent use of latex condoms. This realization embarrassed Dr. Dunn because he had only recently suggested that Clark wear latex condoms during sexual intercourse, an invitation to a life-threatening allergic reaction. Additionally, Dr. Dunn considered how Clark's occupation as an anesthesiologist could contribute to his wife's allergic reaction. During anesthesia, Clark frequently wore cornstarch-powdered latex gloves to protect him and his patients from contact with disease-causing bacteria and viruses. With all of the frequent glove changes at work between patients, Clark's hair skin and clothes became coated each day with cornstarch that flew off of the glove surfaces. This cornstarch carried the latex proteins and acted as a vehicle for transfer of the allergy-causing latex proteins within the hospital and his home. Dr. Dunn shared with Linda and Clark his feeling that he was close to identifying the source of her allergic reaction, natural rubber latex. He promised them that he would undertake a series of diagnostic tests to test this hypothesis. A sample of Linda's blood was collected to send to an outside laboratory for a latex sensitivity test.

Dr. Dunn told them that certain fatalities in the past almost invariably occurred among undiagnosed and unsuspecting latex-allergic patients who were exposed to latex during medical procedures. He explained that a latex-sensitive patient has an allergic response to several proteins present in the rubber tree from which latex is harvested; these proteins remain in latex products like gloves, balloons, condoms, and dental dams after processing and manufacture. Even a minuscule amount of the latex proteins can trigger life-threatening reactions in exquisitely sensitive patients.

Linda listened carefully but was still visibly confused. "While I think I understand what you've said so far, I'm bewildered by the fact that most of my reactions have occurred when I'm nowhere near a latex glove or anything else made of latex," she said. Dr. Dunn thought for a moment before he answered her puzzling question. "Yes, your case illustrates a very interesting phenomenon with latex allergy," the allergist said. "And this is where Clark can help me help you. You are probably being exposed to the latex indirectly through Clark."

Dr. Dunn explained that the latex proteins in latex gloves can become absorbed by the powder that is often on the surface of the gloves. When powdered latex gloves are put on or removed, the protein-containing powder is liberated from the surface of the gloves, becomes airborne, and then drifts down to settle wherever it lands. Consequently, Dr. Dunn asserted, it was very likely that the proteins remained on Clark's hands from the gloves he used, and that the protein-containing powder from the gloves used by all members of the operating room staff remained on the skin of Clark's arms and face, his mustache, and perhaps, on his clothes and shoes.

Linda was instructed to avoid latex exposure by refraining from any bodily contact with her husband until he removed all hospital clothing, showered, and donned a clean set of clothing after work daily. Dr. Dunn suggested that this clothing change as well as showering occur in an isolated bathroom that Linda should not access. Dr. Dunn also suggested that Clark use powder-free gloves at work to minimize airborne transfer of the latex proteins to his face, hair, and clothes. Dunn insisted that Linda learn the long list of medical and consumer products that contain latex and that she faithfully avoid contact with them as natural rubber latex could trigger a fatal allergic reaction. Rubber products were not safe for Linda. He stressed that Clark would now have to avoid using latex condoms, noting that there were new polyurethane condoms available on the market. From a bulletin entitled, "Latex Allergy News," (Torrington, CT) he xeroxed a list of latex-free products that she could use daily. He also suggested that Linda carry latex-free examination gloves for any medical or dental appointments and gave her a box of powder-free vinyl examination gloves to take home with her.

Linda's blood test revealed that she was latex-sensitive, leading Dr. Dunn to reiterate the life-threatening risks of latex exposure and the need to carry an emergency epinephrine kit at all times. He also strongly recommended that Linda immediately order a Medic-Alert bracelet to wear at all times.

Both Linda and Clark developed a new knowledge of the abundant uses of rubber. From tennis shoes to balloons, latex was everywhere. If Linda ever returned to work, she would need to find a nursing environment that permitted only the use of powder-free gloves by her coworkers. She, herself, would be restricted to nonlatex gloves.

The conversion to a latex-free home was an enormous, challenging task to which Linda and Clark were committed. As they changed their home environment, they developed a new sense of freedom that Linda's life was safe. This life-saving benefit was weighed against an obvious sense of social isolation because their world, including the hospital, was filled with natural latex products. At work, Clark switched to using a brand of gloves that was powder-free with a lower content of allergy-provoking latex proteins. To his chagrin, he was unsuccessful in convincing all members of the operating room staff to convert to using powder-free gloves. Clark's new practice of changing clothes, bathing and dressing in a separate bathroom eliminated many of Linda's allergic skin reactions, yet Linda still reported occasional facial rashes after kissing and hugging her husband.

Concerned about his inability to convince his colleagues to convert to the use of powder-free gloves with low levels of latex proteins, Clark discussed this problem with the Chief of Anesthesiology, Dr. Paul Root. Because he had a long and amiable professional association with his boss for more than 10 years, Clark thought that he would support his efforts for a powder-free operating room. Dr. Root began the meeting by saying that he was saddened by Linda's long ordeal, but he was glad that Dr. Dunn has found the cause of her problem and identified a solution. He realized that Clark had asked the operating room personnel to use powder-free gloves. Dr. Root continued by saying that he had contacted the purchasing department, requesting that they consider the possibility of purchasing only powder-free gloves for the operating room. Because powder-free gloves cost nearly twice that of powdered gloves, it would nearly double the cost for surgical gloves in this hospital. The head of the purchasing department estimated that it would cost an additional $75,000 per year. Dr. Root ended by saying that, in a day of managed care and cost containment in our hospital environment, these costs are exorbitant and cannot presently be absorbed by the hospital; therefore, the hospital could not convert to a powder-free operating room. He assured Clark that he would reconsider the possibility of converting to powder-free gloves if the financial situation of the hospital would improve.

Clark was shocked by the well-prepared monologue of his colleague and friend, and by Dr. Root's adversarial posture based on calculated financial costs rather than on healthcare issues. As Clark turned to leave the office, he felt he had been pressured to join a conspiracy of silence.

Virginia's Story

Virginia awoke from her fourth operation to see a bouquet of brightly colored cardboard flowers on her bedstand. The loving note accompanying the beautiful hand-crafted daisies brought tears to her eyes as she thought of her vibrant, thoughtful sons, whom she longed to hold. Although the supportive environment of the Woodrow Wilson Hospital had always felt nurturing to her, Virginia immediately started counting the minutes until she could again be free of the hospital, free to return home to try to reconstruct her personal and professional life.

Virginia got her wish three days later when she was welcomed back into her warm Greenwhich Village home and the embrace of her husband, her children, and her loving extended family. Emotionally drained and physically tender from her recent surgery, she needed the comfort invariably provided by a familiar environment and her husband Bob, and by their circle of close friends who dissipated the recurrent feelings of hopelessness that plagued her multiple times each day. When Virginia returned for her postoperative appointment with Dr. Thomas, she did so with renewed inner strength.

Dr. Thomas had interesting news for Virginia and Bob. "This pathology report is very significant," Dr. Thomas said handing them the paper. "The pathologists found an irritant in the center of your adhesions." He went on to explain the rest of the report. The pathologist indicated that Linda's adhesions were formed predominantly of fibrous tissue, like that found in all other adhesions; but her adhesions contained collections of cornstarch powder particles surrounded by evidence of an inflammatory response that consisted of numerous white cells interspersed between a network of collagen strands that formed the structural components of adhesions. The cornstarch powder particles in Virginia's adhesions were similar to the powder particles applied by manufacturers to the surface of the surgical gloves used in surgery. Surrounding the cornstarch particles were cells that her body recruited to protect against foreign substances, the same types of cells that are also designed to fight microorganisms, like bacteria and viruses.

Medical science allowed the pathologist two different ways to distinguish cornstarch in Virginia's tissues; both involved the examination of the tissue under a microscope. In the first method, the pathologist placed the adhesion sample in a glass slide and rinsed it with a specific dye to stain the tissue. A Periodic Acid Schiff (PAS) stain, a standard dye, was first used to examine Virginia's surgical specimen. The PAS stained the cornstarch particles fuchsia, easy to see among the rest of the light pink fibrous tissue and the light pink and blue inflammatory cells. The fuchsia indicated that the particles were starch, but the pathologist could not distinguish if they were plant or animal starch. The doctor next used a special solution containing iodine on a sample of Virginia's adhesions, a technique that caused the small particles of plant starch to turn black. Because plant starch is the only type of substance that blackens when exposed to the iodine solution, the cornstarch particles in Virginia's adhesions were identified as black spots in otherwise pink fibrous tissue.

The second method used by the pathologist was an examination of Virginia's adhesions under the microscope using a special kind of illumination; this method was necessary to determine that the plant starch particles derived from corn plants. In a normal ray of light, the transverse vibrations of light energy occur in all planes; cornstarch in an unstained tissue sample of an adhesion would be invisible with a normal ray of light. Polarized light is special because all of the rays of light energy are oriented only in one plane. Cornstarch is easily identified when the pathologist uses polarized light microscopy; the particles appear as bright crystals with a Maltese-cross shape. The Maltese-cross shape is seen only if the starch crystals are made of cornstarch. These Maltese cross-shaped crystals were evident throughout Virginia's adhesions.

"The body often attacks foreign substances, and an inflammatory reaction results," Dr. Thomas said. "Although it is rare, some people mount a strong inflammatory reaction when powder particles are shed from surgical gloves and left in the tissues. This process is called a 'foreign body reaction.' The pathologist has given us very strong evidence that your adhesions were caused by a strong foreign body reaction. This inflammatory reaction was directed against the powder coating the surgical gloves that we used during the surgery for your ovarian cyst, and that we have used in each of your subsequent surgeries. Yours is a rare condition, Virginia, but one that we can prevent in the future," he concluded.

As he finished speaking, Bob and Virginia could see that Dr. Thomas seemed almost pleased to offer this new insight into her painful, recurrent illness. Virginia still felt shocked. "Why didn't they figure this out before?" she asked. "I can't believe I had to go through surgery three additional times before we discovered that each time, you were, in a way, propagating the problem!" Dr. Thomas replied, "I asked that question too. It turns out that any cornstarch left behind is usually absorbed into your body three months after your surgery. This is good news and bad news. The good news is that its ability to elicit inflammation does not persist after the three months. The bad news is that if we look for glove powder in the surgical specimen from your adhesions, we may not find any cornstarch particles after three months, but the damage has been done. While cornstarch remains in your tissues, the powder will continue to promote adhesion formation. Once it is absorbed, the adhesions will not become worse, but neither will they diminish. Because your last operation for intestinal obstruction caused by adhesions occurred within three months of your previous operation for release of adhesions causing intestinal obstruction, our pathologists were able to identify the cornstarch particles. In previous procedures, the time interval exceeded 12 months and the pathologists were not able to identify the cornstarch particles in those adhesions that caused intestinal obstruction."

Virginia then asked, "During my last operation, did you wear gloves coated with cornstarch?" "Yes I did," he said, "but I made every effort to wash the cornstarch from the glove surface before surgery." Virginia, unsatisfied with his response, asked, "Well, didn't you wash the cornstarch from your gloves before the first three operations?" Dr. Thomas replied, "Of course I did. I always wash the cornstarch from my gloves before performing surgery. Recent scientific studies suggest that some individuals may be 'hypersensitive' to cornstarch and react with an exaggerated inflammatory response to the glove powder." When Virginia asked if there were surgical gloves without powder, he responded affirmatively, "Yes, there are powder-free gloves, but the cost of powder-free gloves is twice as expensive as that of powdered gloves. In this day of managed care and cost containment, hospitals are reluctant to purchase powder-free gloves for all of our patients." Bob asked if sets of powder-free gloves for patients like Virginia could be ordered in the event of additional surgery. Dr. Thomas smiled with some relief at Bob's question. "I have already ordered powder-free gloves for my surgical team to be used in any future surgical procedure."

At this point, Virginia decided to end the interrogation. She had become a partner in a conspiracy of silence. While she would now have to wait for the next colicky signs of recurrent intestinal obstruction, she was consoled that she would at least gain the benefit of having her own surgery for this recurrent intestinal obstruction performed with powder-free gloves. Still, she wondered who would protect the other patients in the hospital.

Peter's Story

When Dr. Campbell's telephone call was transferred into Peter's office, Peter started talking immediately. "Dr. Campbell, I have a lump below the site of my operation, and I think I have cancer. I need your help."

Dr. Campbell realized the urgency of Peter's cry for help and said she would meet him in two hours in Dr. Richard Smith's office. In the examination room, Dr. Smith carefully pressed his fingertips near the swelling and detected the hard two-centimeter mass beneath the incision that appeared to be without any evidence of inflammation. This finding puzzled Dr. Smith, who believed that the swelling was most likely due to a blood clot in the wound. Although he thought that this nontender mass would disappear spontaneously, he believed that Peter's fears of cancer could be relieved only by microscopic examination of a biopsy of the swelling. Dr. Smith told Peter that he wanted to take a sample of the tissue, a procedure that would easily be performed in his office under local anesthesia. He planned to send the biopsy sample to the pathologist who could tell with certainty through microscopic examination the reason for the swelling and return the results to Peter in two days.

After putting on his mask and surgical gloves, Dr. Smith washed the skin overlying the mass with a brownish solution containing an antiseptic agent. The site of the surgical skin incision was then anesthetized using local anesthesia. After the surgeon deepened the incision through the skin, a fibrotic mass of tissue filled with traces of a brown material resembling dried blood became readily apparent. The fibrous mass had no obvious, well-developed blood supply and was easily removed from the wound with the handle of the scalpel. Because there was no visible sign of infection, Dr. Smith closed the incision with two monofilament nylon sutures. The removed tissue mass was placed in a formalin jar and sent to the pathologist's office. Dr.

Smith promised to meet with Peter to discuss the results of the pathologist's report.

Two days later, Peter arrived expectantly at Dr. Smith's office, somehow anticipating the worst news, cancer. As Peter sat in a comfortable chair across from Dr. Smith's desk, he said, "Well, tell me the bad news."

Dr. Smith smiled. "It's only good news, Peter. First, it was not cancer. It was a granuloma, an abnormal collection of tissue composed of fibrin from blood clots, connective tissue from scarring, and many white cells. Interspersed between the connective tissue strands was foreign material that the pathologist has identified as cornstarch granules." Peter was quite surprised and asked, "How do you use cornstarch in surgery?"

Dr. Smith responded, "Cornstarch is used to coat surgical gloves. Cornstarch powder acts as a lubricant to release the glove from the manufacturing mold, and also helps surgeons slide the gloves on more easily during surgery. Despite the efforts of the surgical team to remove cornstarch from the glove surface, some of the particles remain on the glove and inadvertently get into the wound. These cornstarch particles can result in an inflammatory response and the formation of abnormal tissue called a granuloma. Because the cornstarch is absorbed within three months, the granulomas will usually disappear. Because of your concern about cancer, I thought it was important to identify with certainty the cause of the swelling and allay your fears."

Dr. Smith went on to say that in his 20 years of surgical practice, he had encountered only four such cases of cornstarch granulation that necessitated reoperation. He then pointed to his collection of medical textbooks. "I believe that only 100 cases have been reported in the world literature during the last 50 years since cornstarch use began." He said that powder-free gloves are available, but they are twice as expensive as those with cornstarch, and granuloma formation from cornstarch does not happen that often. He promised that, if Peter ever required additional surgery, he would use surgical gloves without cornstarch. The agreement between Peter and Dr. Smith is a joint pact that becomes a fundamental part of the conspiracy of silence.

Jack and Renee's Story

Once again Jack and Renee entered the soothing decor of Dr. Blake's office. Armed with a renewed sense of hope, the couple was ready for answers. Renee, still weak and tender from her recent operation, held onto Jack's arm for balance as they approached the receptionist. Renee was ushered into an examination room so that Dr. Blake could assess that she was convalescing properly. As he watched the couple enter his office, Dr. Blake considered the emotional impact these months had taken on Renee. She did not seem to have the same enthusiastic glow in her eye that was present at their initial visits. After a brief examination, Dr. Blake invited Jack and Renee to join him in his office to discuss the results of the pathology report from the last operation.

Dr. Blake stated, "Renee, Jack, I have some interesting news for you." He handed the pathology report to Renee. The report was very significant. The pathologists found an irritant in the center of her adhesions. Renee handed the pathology report to Jack as she listened intently to Dr. Blake's words. Dr. Blake continued to explain the remainder of the pathologists' report. The pathologists found that, in addition to the predominant fibrous tissue found in adhesions of most infertility patients, Renee's adhesions also contained collections of cornstarch powder particles surrounded by evidence of inflammation caused by the particles. He went on to explain that the pathologist, using polarized light microscopy, determined that the particles were cornstarch. This technique easily identifies cornstarch particles as brightly illuminated crystals with a Maltese-cross shape. These Maltese-cross shapes were present throughout all of the adhesions around Renee's ovary.

Dr. Blake continued, "Cornstarch is commonly used to coat the surface of surgical gloves. It is a lubricating substance that helps surgeons don the gloves before and during the procedures. It is most likely that the cornstarch was introduced into the wound created during your emergency appendectomy three months ago. Research has shown that cornstarch left in a patient's body is absorbed three months after surgery. Its ability to elicit inflammation does not persist after the three months. If we had waited any longer to release your adhesions, we would not have been able to decipher the cause of the inflammatory response that led to the formation of these adhesions." When Renee asked, "If this cornstarch causes these adhesions which are keeping me from having a baby, why don't they make gloves without cornstarch?" Dr. Blake replied, "As a matter of fact, Renee, powder-free gloves are available; however, powder-free gloves are twice as expensive as the powdered ones. The hospital is under severe financial constraints, and in this era of managed care and cost containment, it is virtually impossible to purchase these gloves for use on all of our patients. We use them routinely in infertility cases, but they are not available for emergency general surgery cases." Jack was frustrated by this response and blurted out another question. "How much more does a powder-free glove cost than a glove covered by powder?" Dr. Blake was bewildered because he did not have an exact answer to the question. "Jack, I am not sure of the difference in cost between a powdered glove and a powder-free glove because gloves are purchased by the purchasing department of the hospital."

Renee asked about her chances of having a baby and was worried about the adhesions coming back. Dr. Blake informed the couple that the adhesions that he recently removed would not reform once the cornstarch was absorbed into the body and was not present to generate an inflammatory response. She and Jack asked Dr. Blake if he wore powdered gloves when he separated Renee's adhesions ten days ago. Dr. Blake answered, "For all infertility surgery, the operating room staff uses only powder-free gloves. In fact, the operating rooms in the Department of Obstetrics and Gynecology are all powder-free. Consequently, I still feel optimistic that Renee will have a baby. If you are unsuccessful in conceiving a child, I can assure you that I will try more sophisticated techniques like in vitro fertilization or, if desired, will facilitate any planned adoption applications. I want to emphasize that there is still a real possibility that Renee is fertile and will conceive a child after her recent laparoscopic surgery. Consequently, I feel very optimistic for your future."

Dr. Blake stated that he had written a letter to the head of the operating room committee expressing his concerns about the use of powdered surgical lubricants on gloves. The head of the operating room committee called and promised that he would survey the entire surgical staff to ask if they would consider using powder-free gloves. If the surgeons agreed to change to the use of powder-free gloves, he would then request the purchasing department to convert to a powder-free operating room environment. He went on to say that purchasing decisions would also have to be approved by the hospital's chief executive officer who administrates the budget.

Jack listened patiently as he considered how the massive medical bureaucracy smothered decision-making and empathized with Dr. Blake's plight. Jack thanked Dr. Blake and said how much he and Renee appreciated his devoted support. Jack and Renee left the office as partners in a conspiracy of silence.

Jim's Story

Dr. Fedson placed one portion of the aspirate from the sterile syringe into a culture tube that would grow bacteria in the presence or absence of oxygen. The remainder of the needle aspirate was sent in a sterile tube to the pathology department. Because Dr. Fedson felt that the endophthalmitis was caused by a bacterial infection, she recommended emergency culturing of the aspirate in the microbiology department and decided that the examination of the aspirate by the pathologist could be delayed this late Friday afternoon until Monday morning. Dr. Fedson assured Jim that she believed that a bacterial infection caused the endophthalmitis and that his condition would respond to an antibiotic administered intravenously. Realizing the urgency of this potentially blinding ophthalmic infection, she admitted Jim to the hospital to be treated with a broad spectrum antibiotic that could easily easily penetrate the tissue of his eye. Jim resigned himself to remain at bed rest with his head positioned on two pillows.

The preliminary results of the bacteriology report gave no comfort to Dr. Fedson or Jim; the result proved sterile, revealing no bacteria. Dr. Fedson had expected an earlier detection of bacteria. She explained to Jim that some bacteria that grow in the absence of oxygen cannot be identified until 72 hours after the specimen has been cultured. Realizing that his endophthalmitis could be caused by a relatively unusual type of bacteria, she broadened the antibiotic treatment to include one that effectively killed anaerobic bacteria (bacteria that grew in the absence of oxygen) in the eye.

The following 48 hours were the longest 48 hours of Jim's life as he waited expectantly for some resolution of the redness and swelling of his inflamed eye. Unfortunately, the inflammation persisted without improvement in his vision. As Jim saw Dr. Fedson each day, he could detect a despondence and disappointment in her voice as she indicated that the culture results were negative, revealing no bacterial growth.

On Monday morning, Dr. Fedson received an urgent call from the Department of Pathology. Dr. Richard Phelps had detected an unusual foreign material within the specimen sent to his laboratory. On microscopic examination using polarized light, Dr. Phelps saw numerous Maltese crosses that were consistent with the diagnosis of cornstarch contamination. Dr. Phelps came quickly to the point, "Dr. Fedson, how did cornstarch get into your patient's eye?" She reflected on the operative procedure and responded, "The only thing I can think of is the cornstarch on my surgical gloves; however, I wash the cornstarch off with wet gauze sponges before performing surgery. Moreover, I try to use a no-touch technique with my gloves so that only my instruments contact the patient's eyes."

Dr. Phelps recommended that she start treating Jim immediately with corticosteroids in an effort to suppress this inflammatory response. The specimen should have been examined earlier so that treatment with the antinflammatory agents could have begun. Delayed treatment of endophthalmitis caused by cornstarch may be ineffective. Dr. Fedson called the charge nurse to initiate the administrate of systemic corticosteroids, cancelling her previous order for antibiotics. The steroids were administered immediately before Dr. Fedson could interrupt her busy office hours to speak to her frightened patient. When she arrived at the hospital, she tried to put a positive emphasis on the recent pathologic findings. "Jim, I'm delighted that we found the cause of the severe inflammation of your eye. It appears to be due to an irritant called cornstarch. The cornstarch used by families in caring for babies is the same material used to powder the surfaces of surgeons' gloves. This dusting powder helps us put on the gloves during surgery. If the cornstarch was not there, surgeons would have a difficult time using surgical gloves. Knowing that cornstarch is a potential irritant, I carefully remove it from the outer surface of my gloves by washing them with a wet cloth.

Because cornstarch produces an inflammatory reaction, I'm treating you with an anti-inflammatory drug, a steroid, which should suppress the inflammatory reaction of the powder in your eye. I plan to continue to administer the drug to you in your veins over the next four days, after which you can take this drug by mouth until the inflammation disappears and you regain your sight."

Jim hoped that the puzzle had been solved and a treatment found that would allow him to see again. He expected that the anti-inflammatory drug would reduce the degree of inflammation, allowing him at least the same level of visual acuity that he enjoyed before surgery. Worried that he might need additional surgery, he asked Dr. Fedson if it was necessary to surgically remove the cornstarch from his eye. She assured him that this would not be necessary because cornstarch was an absorbable powder that would disappear in three months.

Many of Dr. Fedson's promises came true. The anti-inflammatory drug considerably relieved the inflammation in Jim's eye. The redness, swelling, and fluids within his eye gradually disappeared. However, this disappearance of inflammation was not associated with a dramatic improvement in his visual acuity. By three months, his ability to see with his left eye had worsened to 20/200. Jim's hopes for driving a car, reading a newspaper, and singing in the choir had disappeared. He experienced increasing social isolation. Jim continued to see Dr. Fedson, who provided some emotional support to Jim. She identified him as the only case of endophthalmitis she had ever experienced. While such an acknowledgment may have been comforting to other patients, it was not so for Jim, who experienced deep sadness daily. Other elderly friends who experienced successful cataract surgery offered no consolation to Jim as he watched them drive their cars safely throughout the community. When he asked one of his closest friends who had undergone successful cataract surgery the powerful question, "Why me?", his friend suggested that he seek the advice of another ophthalmologist to better understand his complicated and disheartening journey with cataract surgery.

For a second opinion he went to a prestigious university hospital where he was informed that his endophthalmitis was indeed caused by cornstarch on his surgeon's gloves. He found that this severe complication could have been prevented by his surgeon's wearing powder-free surgical gloves. While they could offer him no hope for surgical improvement in his left eye, he was asked to consider cataract surgery on his right eye. This news angered Jim considerably because he was unaware that powder-free gloves were available and that his surgical complication could have been prevented. Moreover, he had lost confidence in Dr. Fedson, who, he felt, did not take adequate responsibility for this complication of eye surgery. He decided not to personally confront Dr. Fedson, preferring to seek legal counsel regarding the merits of his complaints. A friend referred Jim to an attorney who specialized in malpractice claims. After careful review of Jim's operative records and the second opinion from the ophthalmologist at University Hospital, Jim's attorney felt that his complaints were justified and provided grounds for litigation that would end a conspiracy of silence. His attorney filed complaints against the glove manufacturer, the hospital, and Dr. Fedson. The attorneys representing the insurance carriers for the defendants agreed to a settlement out of court for an undisclosed amount of money with the provision that the defendants had no admission of liability and with an agreement that the amount of the settlement would not be disclosed by any party. Although Jim would have preferred the public to be adequately warned about the dangers of dusting powders, he and his attorney decided to settle the case out of court because of their fears of the cost of prolonged litigation. While their decision is understandable, they ultimately joined the conspiracy of silence because their malpractice litigation will not be part of any public record.

———

After writing each of the narrative descriptions of the five fictionalized stories in this chapter, I felt I had developed a deep personal attachment to each of the individuals. A physician develops an intimate bonding with the patient in which they join as inseparable partners in the patient's journey toward recovery. Regardless of the severity of an individual case, I can assure you that I become emotionally involved in the outcome. When my patient developed a complication following surgery, I always viewed it as an error in my judgment that would be corrected in any future surgery. I try to explain to the patient my role in contributing to the complication as well as my planned efforts to correct the problem. As the patient faced emotional frustration and pain associated with the complication, I must admit that I suffered with them during the journey to complete recovery. Often I have developed deep, lasting friendships with these patients that were extended over decades.

The search for the culprit that causes the illness or complication is an important lesson for the physician and patient. This revelation should be acknowledged and celebrated by the patient and healthcare giver. After realizing that the recurrent disease can be prevented, the health professional is faced with an additional responsibility of preventing this complication from developing in other patients. This quest for disease or complication prevention is just as important and exciting as the search for the cause. Sometimes, moreover, the fragility of the souls of some health professionals makes it difficult for them to change the world.

CHAPTER THREE

Latex Allergy Epidemic

"What a long and protracted search it was, and how simple in the end its solution."

Dr. Owen H. Wangensteen

During the last hundred years, latex products have become ubiquitous in our environment. Latex is used in more than 40,000 medical, industrial, and household products, ranging from surgical gloves to sneakers. Latex's popularity can be attributed to its unique performance characteristics, which include strength, elasticity, tear resistance, and superior barrier qualities. Natural rubber latex is harvested from the sap of the commercial rubber tree, *Havea brasiliensis* (Figure 3.1). This sap is a complex mixture containing particles of rubber dispersed in a waterlike liquid. Natural latex contains 2 percent to 3 percent protein. Of the 240 types of proteins found in rubber, 60 show reactivity with antibodies from latex-allergic patients. Because many similar proteins are found in different plants and foods, cross-allergies between latex and different foods, such as bananas, avocados, and kiwi, have been reported frequently.

The vast majority of *Havea brasiliensis* cultivation occurs in Malaysia, Indonesia, and Thailand. After latex is harvested by sap collection from the rubber tree, ammonia is added immediately to prevent bacterial contamination and clumping of the

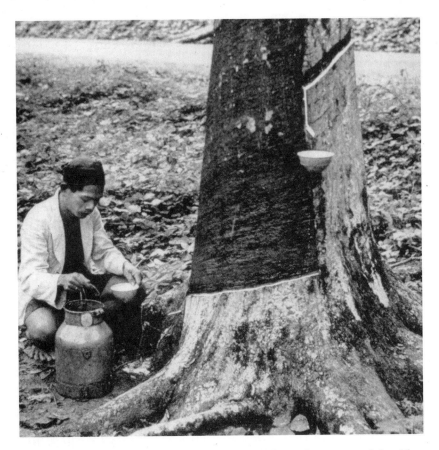

Figure 3.1 A planatation worker collects sap from the commercial rubber tree and empties it into a large metal container.

latex (Figure 3.2). The collected latex is later concentrated by centrifugation to remove water. Manufacturers of rubber products add chemicals, called accelerators, antioxidants, and secondary preservatives, to the concentrated latex preparations, ultimately altering the processing and properties of the finished latex products.

Approximately 90 percent of the harvested rubber is used in the manufacture of extruded rubber products (e.g., rubber thread), injection molded goods (e.g., rubber seals, diaphragms), or automobile tires. The remaining 10 percent of the harvested rubber is used in the manufacture of dipped products, including rubber gloves, condoms, and balloons. Dipped products appear to be responsible for most of the allergic reactions to natural rubber latex.

Two basic techniques of dipping are used in the production of latex gloves and condoms. Surgical and industrial gloves are most often created by coagulant dipping, which involves the use of a salt deposited on the porcelain hand-shaped mold (former). These porcelain formers hang from a continuous, automated production line, passing through various chemicals. The formers then dip repeatedly into latex, after which they are heat-cured by oven-drying. Straight dipping techniques, used for the production of very thin films like condoms and examination gloves, involve the use of formers dipped directly into the latex compound (without the use of salt). The thin latex film is then oven-dried. Once the coagulant or straight dipping step is complete, the oven-dried gloves are passed through water tanks to remove water-soluble proteins and any excess additives. Gloves are then cured by vulcanization, a heated process in which the latex particles become cross-linked in the presence of sulfur.

Some manufacturers then add medicine's deadly dust, cornstarch, applying it to the finished glove surface. This deadly dust is applied to ease removal from the porcelain former and aid surgeons in donning the gloves in the operating room. Other manufacturers process powder-free gloves by coating their surfaces with a gel or by passing the gloves through a chlorine wash that makes the glove surface more slippery. The chlorine wash makes the surface slicker so the gloves are easier to put on. In addition, the wash reduces the amount of allergy-causing protein in the glove. After these processing steps, the powdered and powder-free gloves are stripped from their formers and packaged for distribution.

Most scientists agree that the allergy-causing latex particles are present in raw rubber tree sap and persist in finished latex

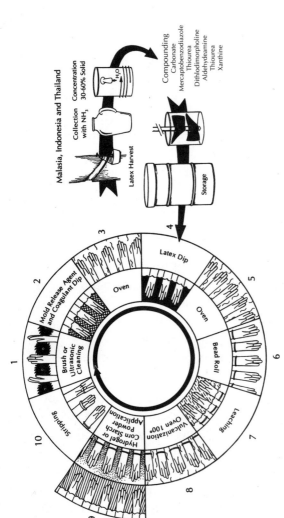

Figure 3.2 The manufacturing process for natural rubber latex gloves. Latex is harvested from the sap of the commercial rubber tree, *Hevea brasiliensis*. Destruction of the latex because of bacterial contamination is prevented by the addition of ammonia to the collected sap. The latex is then concentrated by centrifugation to 30 percent to 60 percent solid. The concentrated latex is then compounded, a process that adds many different chemicals. The latex is shipped and stored until use at glove manufacturing facilities. 1. Production line manufacture starts with the cleaning of porcelain formers attached to a continuous chain. 2. Formers are dipped into a solution containing a mold release agent and a coagulant. 3. The formers coated with the release agent and the coagulant pass through ovens to dry. 4. A dip in the latex produces a uniform rubber film on the formers. 5. The coagulant and heat convert the latex from liquid to solid. 6. A cuff is rolled onto the glove when rotating brushes contact the latex. 7. Single or multiple leaching steps in warm water baths remove excess additives and water-soluble proteins. 8. Heat and sulfur catalyze crosslinking of the latex polymer (vulcanization). 9. Cornstarch is applied as a detackifying agent in powdered gloves. In contrast, application of a hydrogel polymer is used to produce powder-free gloves. 10. Gloves are stripped from the porcelain former.

products. Specifically, the protein components in latex have been incriminated as the agents responsible for latex-specific allergy, with three exceptions. First, the chemical accelerators and antioxidants used in glove manufacture have been long recognized as a cause of irritant reactions (type IV allergic reactions), occurring with the use of latex gloves (that is, dermatitis). Second, when casein, a milk protein, is added as a filler to some brands of surgical and household gloves, it may be responsible for glove-related reactions in milk-sensitive individuals. Third, there are rare reports of allergy to medicine's deadly dust, cornstarch dusting powder, the substance used in most powdered latex gloves.

Scientists have demonstrated that latex proteins are potent allergens capable of inducing potentially fatal allergic reaction. Until recently, accurate measurement of these proteins in latex medical products has proven to be very difficult. Each step of the manufacturing process can be modified to considerably alter the protein fractions in latex. Latex proteins can be divided into three groups: latex-bound protein, water-soluble protein, and starch-bound protein.

Some proteins in latex are physically trapped in the glove. They cannot be removed by washing or using the glove. Consequently, these bound latex proteins do not cause latex allergies. In quantifying exposure, debate remains as to whether one should measure the total protein content of latex products or the fraction of proteins that have, so far, been identified to function as allergy-causing particles. Because patients have been shown to recognize many different proteins rather than just a few, measurement of total protein in latex products is now the accepted method of quantifying exposure.

Water-soluble proteins are easily extracted with saline solutions from latex gloves. In 1986, Dr. Teresa Carrillo from Madrid, Spain, and her colleagues first determined that one of the allergy-causing particles in latex was a water-soluble protein. Other investigators later isolated four other water-soluble proteins from latex that seemed responsible for allergic reactions. In the laboratory, these four proteins bound to antibodies in the blood of patients who had experienced life-threatening reactions to latex products. Furthermore, in the office, these four proteins gave positive skin-prick tests in individuals sensitive to latex. Today, over 15 different allergy-causing latex proteins have been identified.

Current investigations indicate that one way of minimizing allergic reactions to latex is removing as much of the water-soluble proteins and irritating manufacturing chemicals as possible from latex products devices. This removal is primarily accomplished by (1) washing processes before and after the heat-curing (vulcanization) step, (2) assuring that washing tanks contain water that is agitated and continuously refreshed to minimize chemical and protein content in the water bath, and (3) immersing the gloves in the washing tanks for an appropriate time. Washing after heat-curing is important because there is evidence that proteins become easier to wash out and move to the surface of latex gloves during heat-curing.

When considering latex allergy, it is also important to note that latex proteins attach to the cornstarch powder. The latex protein-starch particles found on latex gloves represent a potentially reactive allergy-causing particle. Complex antigens, such as those composed of both protein and starch components, have been shown to stimulate the immune system to a greater degree than highly purified antigens. Consequently, the addition of cornstarch to surgical and medical examination gloves during manufacture is thought to create a new set of hazardous latex particles that are even more effective in triggering allergic responses. Moreover, in 1992, Drs. Donald H. Beezhold and William C. Beck of the Guthrie Foundation in Sayer, Pennsylvania, warned that this significant interaction between latex proteins and cornstarch powders not only exacerbated allergy but also promoted the development of latex sensitization.

Up to 700 mg of powder may be on a pair of sterile surgical gloves. The soluble latex proteins on the glove bind to the powder granules, allowing them to be easily deposited on the skin, mucous membrane, or wound. When gloves are donned and removed, this powder-antigen complex flies into the atmosphere, entering the lungs and open wounds. Out of all healthcare workers affected by latex allergy, it has been estimated that 90 percent became latex-allergic because of cornstarch powder.

When healthcare providers put on and remove surgical and medical examination gloves, the starch powder particles with their attached protein easily become airborne and can be inhaled over a period of many hours. Latex-sensitive patients, who inhale these latex protein-cornstarch particles, suffer severe allergic reactions. In addition, because it is very difficult, costly, and time-consuming to remove cornstarch from surgical gloves by washing, surgeons often deposit these protein-coated starch particles in wounds.

Research shows that, immediately after powdered glove removal, considerable protein remains on the hand of the glove-wearer. Protective hand creams applied before donning of surgical gloves actually increased the amount of latex protein transferred from gloves to the hands of the wearers. Further, it was shown that powder-free gloves transferred little to no measurable protein

Before 1996, the Food and Drug Administratrion (FDA) indicated that a certain group of gloves could be labeled "hypoallergenic." This term, "hypoallergenic," referred only to the content of chemicals in the gloves that caused skin irritation and dermatitis and did not refer to the latex proteins that cause life-threatening systemic reactions. Overall, gloves labeled "hypoallergenic" tended to have less allergy-causing latex proteins and chemicals than gloves without the "hypoallergenic" designation; however, 11 of the 24 measured lots of "hypoallergenic" gloves had significant amounts of latex protein allergens.

Until recently, complications stemming from the use of latex products were thought to be limited to contact dermatitis, an inflammation of the skin. During the last decade, the prevalence of latex allergy has reached epidemic levels. Today, latex allergy is considered by many to be the largest problem faced by the healthcare profession since the outbreak of the Acquired Immunodeficiency Syndrome (AIDS). While latex allergy is not a recent development, it has only been during the last five years that public health officials have acknowledged its potentially life-threatening consequences and enormous economic costs.

Many allergy experts incriminate the introduction of Universal Precautions in the late 1980s as a major causal factor in the increased frequency of latex-allergic reactions. At that time, the Center for Disease Control and Prevention required that health professionals wear gloves to protect themselves from contact with the blood and secretions of their patients. Since 1987, the frequency of glove usage increased dramatically, currently approaching 10 billion gloves per year (Figure 3.3).

The demand for latex gloves exceeded the production capability of quality manufacturers. Consequently, hospitals purchased a large number of latex gloves from lower quality manufacturers to meet demand. The manufacturing processes used in these gloves did not successfully remove the soluble latex proteins. When the soluble latex protein concentration for the quality manufactured gloves was compared with the cheaper gloves there were dramatic differences in the concentrations of total latex protein. The concentration of latex protein found in the cheaper gloves was nearly 3,000-fold greater than that encountered in gloves manufactured with strict quality control.

It was believed that these cheaper gloves with high concentrations of soluble latex proteins caused allergic reactions in many healthcare workers and patients during the early 1990s. When a healthcare worker wore the cheaper high allergen glove, it was estimated that this one exposure was comparable to that of wearing 3,000 gloves containing low levels of soluble latex

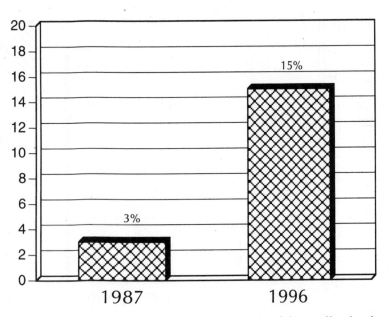

e 3.4 During the last 10 years, the incidence of latex allergies in hcare professionals has increased four-fold and now affects approx-ly 15 percent of healthcare professionals nationwide!

ling of the manufacturing process of latex gloves to under-d best how allergy can be prevented. The allergy-provoking rs in latex can be dramatically reduced by modern techno-advances in latex manufacturing. Today, latex surgical es with low levels of latex allergens should be used exclu-y in medical practice to prevent harm to patients and staff bers.

Groups considered to be at high risk for development of allergy include the following: spina bifida patients, chil-with multiple operative procedures, healthcare workers, allergy patients, and patients with a history of other aller-Patients with spina bifida are at highest risk of developing allergy. Spina bifida is among the most common type of defect. Patients with spina bifida are born with clefts in

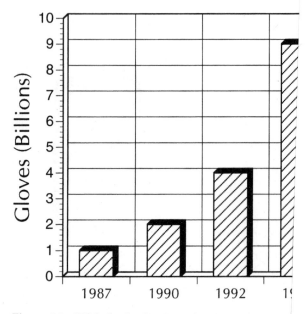

Figure 3.3 With the institution of Universal Precaut
increased from 1 billion pairs per year to 10 billion p

proteins. Despite this revelation of the hig
water-soluble latex proteins in low quality
1980s, these same highly allergenic gloves a
today as routine examination and surgical gl

The FDA had received over 1,100 reports
reactions, including 15 deaths related to the u
ing medical products and devices between
1995, there were over 1,600 reports and 23
allergic reactions to latex. Healthcare worke
the groups exposed to high levels of latex an
at increased risk for the development of la
3.4). Thousands of nurses, doctors, dentists, a
workers jeopardize their health and sac
because of severe latex allergy. Because of th
tions of allergic reactions caused by natur
healthcare professional and consumer must

their spinal column. When multiple levels of the bony spinal column are involved, the saclike membrane covering the spinal cord forms an outpouching that extends through the skin. The severest form of spina bifida is usually associated with severe nerve defects that cause bowel and bladder dysfunction. These patients often experience repeated bladder and kidney infections as well as kidney failure. Physicians who care for infants with severe forms of spina bifida recommend a variety of surgical procedures. Immediately after birth, these patients require surgery to close the skin over the exposed sac covering the spinal cord. Subsequently, each patient often undergoes many other operations to correct bowel and bladder dysfunction, help minimize pain, and correct associated bone and joint problems. During each of these surgical procedures, a child with spina bifida is exposed to many different rubber latex products. Because of the inordinate amount of exposure to different latex products, a great percentage of these children acquire latex allergy.

Dr. Kevin J. Kelly, a noted pediatrician and allergist at the Medical College of Wisconsin, conducted a nationwide study of children's hospitals in 1990. He reported that children with spina bifida had a risk of a life-threatening allergic reaction during surgery that was 500 times greater than that of other children undergoing surgery. He estimated that 40 percent to 65 percent of spina bifida patients were allergic to rubber products. Since his comprehensive report, numerous additional studies have evaluated the risk factors for latex allergy in children with severe forms of spina bifida. All scientists agree that frequent exposure to latex and the presence of other allergies are the two major risk factors for these children.

The pattern of increased risk of latex sensitization associated with multiple surgical procedures is not unique to spina bifida patients. Other patients, who have undergone multiple operations, are also at increased risk for developing latex allergies. In 1993, Dr. Denise-Anne Moneret-Vautrin from France first demonstrated that 6.5 percent of patients, who had undergone multiple operations, were sensitized to latex, while only 0.37 percent of individuals without multiple surgeries or other risk factors were sensitized. A more recent study has shown that children, who have had three or more surgeries, have an incidence of latex allergy as high as 33 percent.

Rubber gloves have been increasingly implicated as the cause of skin irritation, dermatitis, and hives in healthcare workers. In 1987, Dr. Kristina Turjanmaa in the Department of Dermatology, Tampere University Hospital of Finland, was the first to examine the frequency of latex glove allergy among healthcare workers. In that Finnish study, she screened 512 hospital employees using a latex-glove scratch-chamber test. Those employees with a positive scratch-chamber test were then subjected to skin prick tests. Fifteen of the 512 employees (2 percent) had confirmed latex allergy. All latex-allergic personnel could continue their routine work by using a pair of glove liners or by using latex gloves without certain rubber chemicals. Latex glove allergy was significantly more common in operating room personnel than in hospital employees working in examination units and laboratories. In the operating rooms, the latex allergy prevalence was 7.4 percent in physicians, 5.6 percent in nurses, and 5.0 percent in other employees. A study performed in North American hospitals during 1987 demonstrated a remarkably similar prevalence in latex allergy among physicians (9.9 percent vs. 7.4 percent in Finnish physicians).

Dr. I. G. K. Axelsson, of the Department of Thoracic Medicine at the Karalinska Hospital in Stockholm, Sweden, was one of the first to describe an association between latex allergy and food. This physician published a report of a 12-year-old girl who developed an allergic reaction with a runny nose, watery eyes, and itching in the throat after eating stone fruits. Subsequently, she developed allergic swelling of her face and throat after inflating a rubber balloon. More recent studies have demonstrated the existence of a "latex-fruit syndrome," predominantly affecting adult women. These studies confirmed that certain proteins in tropical fruits are similar to those found in latex and may be responsible for latex "cross-reaction" in certain individuals. Latex allergy has now been associated with many fruit allergies to include tomato, grape, pineapple, nuts, figs, passion-fruit, celery, kiwi, citrus fruits, banana, chestnut, avocado, and peach.

Atopy is used to designate a group of individuals who have a personal or family history of one or more of the following diseases: hay fever, asthma, dry skin, and eczema (a red, itchy, scaly inflammation of the skin). The incidence of atopy in the general population approaches 20 percent. In a 1993 study of risk factors for latex allergy, 9.4 percent of atopic patients had latex allergy.

Understanding Allergic Reaction

Under normal circumstances, an individual's immune system responds to an allergy-causing substance, or antigen, such as a latex protein, with a well-controlled inflammatory response. However, damage to a person's tissues and a clinically apparent disease can result from problems with the regulation of any of the components of the immune system. The type of immune response elicited by a foreign antigen is dependent, in part, on the route of exposure to that antigen. Latex absorption through the skin is postulated as the major route of sensitization in healthcare workers. Body sweat inside latex gloves may make latex proteins soluble; the solubilized proteins are then absorbed through the skin, sensitizing the wearer to the latex antigen. Friction, pressure, heat, and perspiration are among the nonspecific factors that influence the occurrence, severity, and sites of involvement of allergic contact dermatitis. Additionally, certain skin diseases predispose to an increased incidence of allergic contact dermatitis. Included among these are eczema, burned skin, and nonspecific irritated skin. Because penetration of the allergen below the top layer of skin is essential for allergenic activity, breaking of the normal skin surface barrier by injury favors sensitization. However, in sensitized individuals, allergen absorption can occur through unbroken skin. When skin exposure occurs, allergic reactions are usually limited to the area of contact, but may progress to other parts of the body.

In addition to direct skin contact, other possible routes of latex sensitization include inhalation, ingestion, surgical procedures, and exposure during passage of tube into a vein, the spine, or other body parts. While exposure to airborne latex allergens in a hospital setting has been well characterized, emerging new data suggest that the risk of sensitization by inhaled allergens may be more widespread. A recent disturbing report in an urban setting observed airborne, irregularly shaped black particles that appeared to represent tire fragments. These observations indicated that latex tire fragments containing latex antigens were abundant in urban air and suggested the possibility that these particles could contribute to latex sensitization and allergy, though this has yet to be confirmed.

Life-threatening allergic response (anaphylaxis) to latex exposure has been shown to occur most commonly during surgery. Anaphylaxis occurred most frequently during abdominal surgery, cesarean sections, and operative procedures on the genitals or urinary tracts. In these situations, the skin barrier was bypassed and latex allergen absorption occurred through the lining of the internal organs.

There are three types of allergic reactions to latex products. The first type is an irritant contact dermatitis. The second is Type IV hypersensitivity, and the third type of allergic reaction is Type I hypersensitivity.

Nonallergic irritant contact dermatitis accounts for 80 percent of all cases of contact dermatitis and occurs when a foreign substance new to the individual causes direct damage to the skin. Chapped skin from hand-washing with detergents is a typical example of a situation capable of producing irritant contact dermatitis. Certain chemicals, such as thiurams, used in the latex manufacture may also cause irritant contact dermatitis. These reactions are very common among individuals who wear latex gloves continually at work. This mild irritant reaction occurs in 25 percent to 40 percent of glove wearers. While these irritant reactions do not involve the immune system, they may be important contributors to allergic reactions to latex.

A Type IV hypersensitivity reaction is a delayed reaction contact dermatitis produced mainly by chemicals added to the latex during its manufacture. While the same chemicals that cause irritant contact dermatitis can produce contact dermatitis (thiuram accelerators 72 percent, carba-mix accelerators 25 percent, mercapto-mix accelerators 3 percent), it must be emphasized that contact dermatitis is a distinct entity involving cells in the immune system. Contact dermatitis consists of two phases: a sensitization, or afferent phase, and later, a trigger, or efferent phase.

The first phase of Type IV hypersensitivity is a sensitization process that involves four steps.

Step 1: A hapten, a small substance that will not generate an immune response on its own, comes in contact with the skin where an antigen presenting cell, typically a Langerhans cell, "traps" the hapten and carries it on one of its surface protein carriers (Figure 3.5). This combination of protein carrier and hapten forms a structure capable of generating an immune response. The Langerhans cell takes in and partially degrades the protein-hapten complex. Protein products of this degradation are brought to the surface of the Langerhans cell.

Step 2: The Langerhans cell with the processed protein on its surface migrates to a regional lymph node (Figure 3.6).

Step 3: The antigen presenting cell (Langerhans cell) presents to a helper T-cell its processed hapten-protein complex on the surface receptor (Figure 3.7). The T-cell becomes sensitized and develops receptors for the particular protein complex combination.

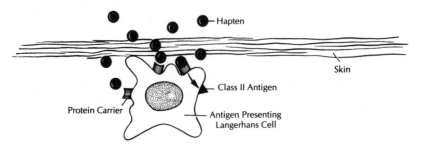

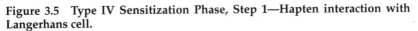

Figure 3.5 Type IV Sensitization Phase, Step 1—Hapten interaction with Langerhans cell.

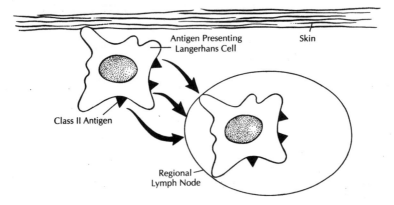

Figure 3.6 Type IV Sensitization Phase, Step 2—Langerhans cell migrates to regional lymph node.

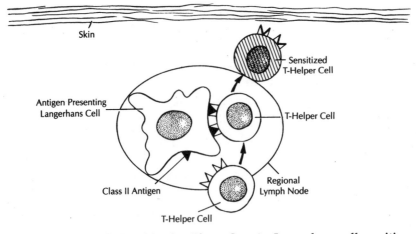

Figure 3.7 Type IV Sensitization Phase, Step 3—Langerhans cell sensitizes T-helper cell.

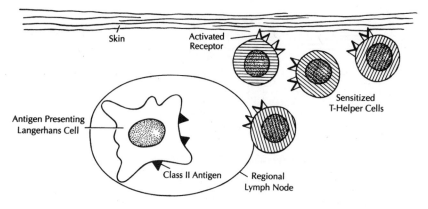

Figure 3.8 Type IV Sensitization Phase, Step 4—Sensitized T-helper cells migrate to the skin.

Step 4: The sensitized T-cell then migrates back to the skin where it serves as an immune system alarm (Figure 3.8).

The second phase of this reaction is a trigger, or efferent, phase that involves three steps.

Step 1: When the sensitized T-cell is subsequently exposed to the same allergen complex, the allergen binds to the cell's receptor. Antigen binding to the sensitized T-cell causes the antigen presenting cell to produce Interleukin 1 (IL-1) (Figure 3.9).

Step 2: IL-1 is a chemical substance that causes T-cells to manufacture and release other chemicals called cytokines and lymphokines. These chemicals include Interleukin 2 (IL-2) and Interferon G (IFN-(); they set off an inflammatory cascade that may activate other parts of the immune system (Figure 3.10).

Step 3: Cells called macrophages in the skin are activated and other inflammatory cells are mobilized. An inflammatory response occurs with the development of increased blood flow and tissue swelling (Figure 3.11). This inflammatory response is recognized as Type IV hypersensitivity. The appearance of this first inflammatory reaction is delayed, occurring at several hours up to four days after reexposure to the chemical, but subsequent

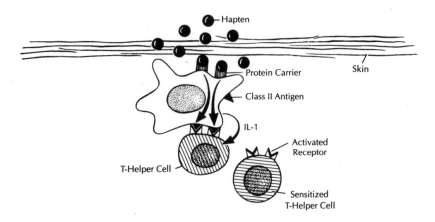

Figure 3.9 Type IV Trigger Phase, Step 1—Processed allergen binds receptor on sensitized T-helper cell causing Langerhans cell to produce IL-1.

reactions develop within a quicker time frame. The tissue swelling and reddened skin are localized initially and can persist for weeks, but ultimately these conditions spread over wider regions. The patient remains sensitized, and an allergic reaction recurs if the individual comes in contact with products containing the same chemical. It is important to note that the development of Type IV hypersensitivity can occur after years of contact

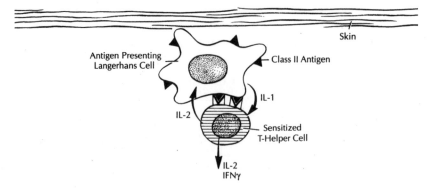

Figure 3.10 Type IV Trigger Phase, Step 2—IL-1 stimulates T-helper cell to produce IL-2 and IFNγ.

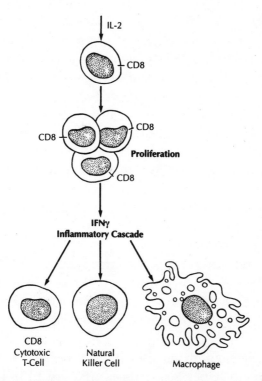

Figure 3.11   Type IV Trigger Phase, Step 3—IL-2 activates cytotoxic T-cells, natural killer cells and macrophages, which cause the Type IV hypersensitivity response.

with a substance. While these Type IV allergic reactions do not become life-threatening, they, like irritant reactions, may predispose the worker to more serious allergic hypersensitivity reactions.

Type I hypersensitivity reactions occur when an antigen interacts with an antibody. This allergic reaction is an immediate reaction that can occur within minutes or at 1 hour to 2 hours after exposure. Type I hypersensitivity reactions can be manifest as localized hives or a life-threatening reaction with involvement of the entire body (systemic reaction). The route of latex antigen presentation will usually dictate the range of symptoms. A patient with skin exposed to the latex allergen will most often first experience skin irritation or hives as a manifestation of allergy, but, in some cases, he or she may initially experience swelling of the face, difficulty breathing and/or life-threatening anaphylaxis. Airborne exposure to latex allergens in sensitized individuals results in severe occupational asthma with eye and nose involvement. Finally, exposure during surgery to latex allergens is the route most often associated with anaphylactic reactions. Generalized hives and swelling of the face and throat (thus limiting breathing) have also been noted to occur during surgery.

Type I hypersensitivity, like Type IV hypersensitivity, consists of two distinct phases: the sensitization, or afferent phase, and the trigger, or efferent phase.

The sensitization process has three steps.

Step 1: An antigen presenting cell, the Langerhans cell, in the skin, the lungs, or the lining of the digestive tract, will first ingest and process the latex protein, which acts as an antigen (Figure 3.12).

Step 2: The Langerhans cell with its processed antigen is then presented to the helper T- and B-cells (Figure 3.13). These T- and B-cells form receptors specific for the processed antigen, becoming sensitized.

Step 3: If latex antigen exposure occurs at the specific receptors on the T- and B-cells, B-cells are induced to begin production of

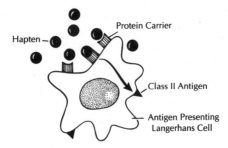

Figure 3.12 Type I Sensitization Phase, Step 1—Hapten interaction with Langerhans cell.

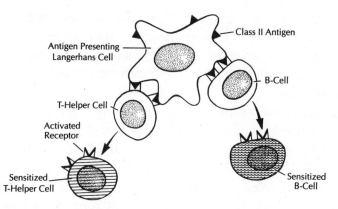

Figure 3.13   Type I Sensitization Phase, Step 2—Langerhans cell sensitizes T-helper cell and B-cell.

latex-specific IgE allergic antibodies (Figure 3.14). This B-cell production of antibody depends on the help of T- helper cells. This sensitization phase may persist for several years and is related to the individual's susceptibility as well as to total latex antigen exposure. The latex-specific IgE antibodies then attach themselves

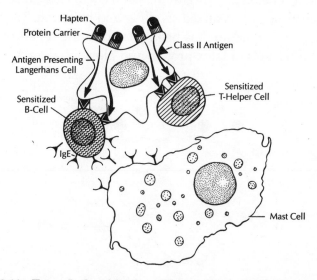

Figure 3.14 Type I Sensitization Phase, Step 3—Processed antigen interacts with sensitized T-helper cells to stimulate B-cell production of IgE.

to receptors on the surface of mast cells, which store chemicals (histamine, serotonin, leukotrienes, etc.) that cause allergic reaction. During this sensitization phase, there is no noticeable illness.

The trigger phase of Type I hypersensitivity occurs on subsequent exposure and involves three steps.

Step 1: The latex antigens react directly with the previously formed latex-specific IgE antibodies found on the surface of mast cells, rather than with the sensitizing B-cells (Figure 3.15).

Step 2: The latex antigen combines with two adjacent antibodies on the mast cell, causing "antigen bridging," an event that initiates a sequence of chemical reactions and a change in the cell membrane (Figure 3.16).

Step 3: The alteration in the cell membrane releases the specific chemical signals characteristic of the Type I hypersensitivity reaction (Figure 3.17). These mediators may be preformed or newly generated. Preformed chemicals released from mast cell granules include histamine and eosinophil chemotactic factor; newly generated signaling chemicals include prostaglandins and leukotrienes. These highly reactive chemicals cause allergic symptoms, such as localized swelling and irritation. The magnitude of allergic reaction has been related to the repetitive exposure to high levels of latex protein and glove powder. When suf-

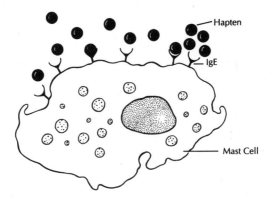

Figure 3.15 Type I Trigger Phase, Step 1—Latex antigen binds to latex specific IgE on mast cell.

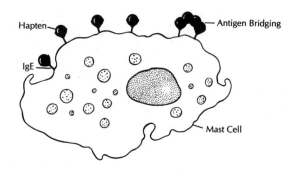

Figure 3.16 Type I Trigger Phase, Step 2—Latex antigen combines with two adjacent antibodies on the mast cell causing antigen bridging.

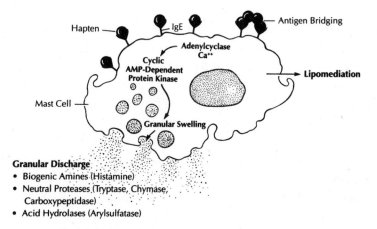

Figure 3.17 Type I Trigger Phase, Step 3—Alteration of mast cell membrane releases mediators of Type I hypersensitivity reaction.

ficient numbers of mast cells are involved, a generalized or anaphylactic reaction will occur.

Signs and Symptoms

While irritant contact dermatitis does not involve the immune system like allergic contact dermatitis, the two can appear similar. With allergic contact dermatitis, the onset of irritant contact dermatitis may be immediate or delayed. Itching is the most common symptom in both the irritant and allergic contact dermatitis. The development of irritant contact dermatitis begins with mild dryness, redness, and scaling. On continued exposure, cracking, crusting, and scaling of the skin may occur. Because the physical features may be so similar with allergic and irritant contact dermatitis, the physician must have an understanding of the patient's exposure to any substances to plan a course to differentiate the two entities.

Type IV hypersensitivity, or allergic contact dermatitis, is based on specific allergic sensitization caused principally by skin contact with the offending agent. Like irritant contact dermatitis, allergic contact dermatitis begins immediately or may be delayed. Likewise, in many cases, the symptoms of allergic contact dermatitis are identical to those of irritant contact dermatitis.

Type I hypersensitivity symptoms separate into four degrees of severity: (1) localized hives; (2) generalized hives with facial and throat swelling; (3) hives with asthma, involvement of the eyes, nose, ears, throat, and digestive tract; and (4) hives with anaphylaxis. With airborne contamination, involvement of the eyes and nose with asthma often predominates. It is becoming evident that some people, especially healthcare workers, progress to long-term asthma and lung disease. It has even been found that some workers develop inflammation of the heart muscle as a result of a long-term immune response syndrome.

Localized hives are the most common early manifestation of rubber allergy, particularly in latex-sensitive healthcare workers. Symptoms appear within 10 minutes to 15 minutes after donning gloves. The raised, reddened wheals that develop are characteristically very itchy. After the hives resolve, no permanent skin discoloration remains.

Episodic runny nose, sneezing, and obstruction of the nasal airway with tearing and widespread itching of eyes, nose, and throat are the primary features of allergic rhinitis. Asthma is characterized by partial obstruction of the airways, which also exhibits excessive secretions, swelling, and inflammation. In long-standing cases, the patient may develop emphysema.

Anaphylaxis has been most commonly encountered during surgery. Also, 15 reported latex allergy associated deaths have been reported during barium enema examinations from exposure to the latex enema tips. It is, however, important to note that anaphylactic reactions have been encountered during gloving, exposure to dental dams and condoms, and even after indirect exposure by contact with individuals who use latex gloves.

The life-threatening anaphylactic response appears within minutes after exposure to the latex antigen. This response is accompanied by severe shortness of breath caused by upper airway obstruction (swelling) and lower airway obstruction (spasm), and is followed by shock. Skin symptoms often occur with anaphylaxis and include itching and hives with or without swelling of the face and throat. Other manifestations include nausea, vomiting, crampy abdominal pain, and diarrhea.

Diagnosis

The diagnosis of latex allergy is made by a careful history and physical examination complemented by laboratory tests (Appendix C). In 1991, the FDA recommended that health professionals screen patients who may have a potential latex allergy, particularly those with severe forms of spina bifida or any patient scheduled for diagnostic or surgical procedures. All physicians are requested to report episodes of anaphylaxis during procedures requiring general anesthesia through state health departments to the Center for Disease Control's National Center for Infectious Disease.

Latex allergy is best diagnosed by talking with the patient and reviewing the detailed history of the illness. Individuals affected by latex allergies often relate similar experiences. Onset often begins almost imperceptibly with dermatitis of the hands, which the patient initially attributes to frequent hand-washing and irritation. After a short period of time (less than a year), redness, blistering, swelling, and itching emerge within one hour to three hours after onset of glove use. For patients presenting with contact dermatitis or hives, location and onset of irritation are important, as are nature of progression and recurrence. Affected healthcare workers often also complain of a history of respiratory symptoms, including rhinitis, recurrent sinus infection, and asthma, pronounced while at work but improved while at home.

Physicians will question such patients about response to over-the-counter medications; history of atopic disease such as asthma, food allergy, anaphylaxis; and hives related to latex contact in the home or community. These questions will help the physician identify patients in groups at high risk of latex-related anaphylaxis. It is important to remember that the majority of reported latex-allergic healthcare workers are employed as physicians, dentists, dental hygienists, and operating room nurses, and have prior histories of contact dermatitis and/or localized hives when using latex gloves. A thorough physical examination must also be performed in order to identify skin, lung, and generalized symptoms of latex allergy.

Currently, diagnosticians have no available "Gold Standard" for the diagnosis of Type I latex allergy, but useful guidelines were recently introduced to evaluate of latex allergy in patients. These guidelines recommend sequential use of blood tests, glove use tests, and skin prick tests to optimize safety and accurate diagnosis. Blood tests should be performed at a reputable laboratory for patients with compelling symptoms. If blood testing is positive, latex allergy is confirmed and no further testing is necessary. If blood testing is negative in a patient in whom latex allergy is strongly suspected, a glove use test should be performed. If the use test is positive, latex allergy is confirmed. If the use test is negative, a skin prick test (using purified latex antigens) is performed as the final diagnostic tool offered. For those physicians performing use testing or skin prick testing, appropriate emergency medical equipment must be available to treat anaphylaxis, a hazard occasionally noted to occur during testing.

Treatment

The first step in patient management is to identify patients who are allergic to latex or are in a high-risk group. The admission form should screen all patients for latex allergy. Patients considered to be at high risk for latex allergy should be classified into the following groups.

- Group 1: Patients with a history of anaphylaxis after exposure to natural rubber latex products.
- Group 2: Patients with a history of contact dermatitis upon exposure to natural rubber latex material.
- Group 3: Patients in the high-risk group without a previous history of latex allergy.

All patients in these three groups should be treated using a latex avoidance protocol in a latex-safe environment (Appendix D). Latex allergy is a serious problem that will only grow in frequency with the passage of time, unless patients demand low allergen, powder-free latex gloves. The time to deal with this epidemic is today, when the problem is still relatively small, and the costs in human suffering and exploding healthcare costs have been significant but not yet devastating. Further procrastinating will only guarantee more suffering and increased costs, not only for hospitals but for society as a whole.

CHAPTER FOUR

Society Awakens

"Many surgeons are great individualists, more likely to rest their arguments upon their own experience, or upon expressions of colleagues known to be friendly to their attitudes, than upon objective evidence. Very rarely did experimental evidence creep into presentations."

Dr. Owen H. Wangensteen

Despite the dramatic life-threatening consequences of latex allergy epidemic, it has not been considered newsworthy, as evidenced by the relative absence of news stories during the long period of this epidemic. When the latex allergy epidemic began to affect large numbers of health professionals in the same hospital house, the latex allergy epidemic was finally judged to be newsworthy, warranting the attention of skilled news reporters.

On Thursday, July 29, 1993, Richard Saltos, a reporter for *The Boston Globe*, wrote an article entitled, "Five Brigham Operating Rooms Close Due to Faulty Ventilation." The article described a mysterious epidemic that sent operating room employees home with headaches and fatigue. This epidemic followed five months of complaints from operating room personnel who reportedly exhibited a wide range of symptoms, including rashes, hives, respiratory irritation, nausea, and heart palpitations. Saltos indicated that, "An internal investigation, which officials say is widening, has traced some of the symptoms to allergic reactions to latex . . . used in surgical gloves and other equipment."

In this same article, Margaret Hanson, clinical vice president of Brigham and Women's Hospital, stated not only that the problem was sapping morale, but also that, on any given day, 12 or 14 operating room employees were unable to work, or were reassigned to desk jobs, because of their allergic reactions. Hanson reported, "None of us are happy about this. People are impatient, and I don't blame them. We all just want to find out what the answer is." Hanson noted that Occupational Safety and Health Administration investigators had visited several times, that environmental experts from the Harvard School of Public Health were looking into the cause of the symptoms, and that nine or ten senior hospital administrators were working on the problem almost full time.

On December 26, 1995, WGBH Educational Foundation aired its NOVA show (#2217) entitled, "Can Buildings Make You Sick?" This insightful documentary detailed the investigation of the "sick-building syndrome" in a variety of different settings and at Brigham and Women's Hospital. Sherwood Burge of the Birmingham Heartlands Hospital, an international expert in health problems caused by buildings, defined the sick-building syndrome as a concurrent set of ". . . very common complaints which are more common in some buildings than in others, and which get better when people go away from that building."

The NOVA documentary provided an update on the Brigham and Women's Hospital where the hospital administration took action after the sick-hospital syndrome worsened during the winter of 1993. Subsequent to closing down the five operating rooms in July 1993, the hospital's administration enlisted the expertise of an environmental consultant, John McCarthy.

McCarthy found that a number of people, who experienced difficulties on the job, developed rashes and also complained of various type of allergic reactions. The affected staff members worked in the operating rooms during shifts that spanned all periods in the day under many different circumstances. It took

McCarthy months of effort to check out an enormous number of potential culprit causes. He searched anything and everything brought into the sterile world of the operating room. After a series of investigations, which involved looking at particles in the air, considering chemicals used in the workplace, examining equipment, and finally, scrutinizing the products used by nurses and physicians in their care of patients, he identified that, for a large number of employees, sensitivity to the latex gloves used in operating rooms caused the sick-building syndrome at Brigham and Women's Hospital.

Unexpectedly, the source of latex exposure was not just from skin contact. When the gloves were donned or removed, medicine's deadly dust used on the glove to aid in glove-donning was released into the air. This dust, it turned out, bound tightly to the allergenic latex proteins and remained airborne for hospital employees to breathe. Each time anyone donned or removed surgical gloves, more powder was liberated into the environment. The powder would lodge itself on the anesthetists' gowns, would form a thin coat covering flat surfaces throughout the room, would fall to the floor where it could later be reaerosolized again and again, and could also be found to adhere electrostatically to surgical sutures and instruments.

Once McCarthy understood the source of the sick-building syndrome, he instituted a vigorous cleaning program for all gurneys, beds, hospital supplies, walls, ceilings, and ventilation system. It took months of meticulous cleansing to remove the powder, but the hardest task was making sure that the latex aeroallergen levels were controlled.

John Gaida, Vice President, Brigham and Women's Hospital, emphasized the magnitude of the problem by pointing out, "Most hospitals could use as many as ten different brands of gloves in their operation, from exam gloves, to surgeons' gloves, to procedure gloves, all different kinds of gloves. We took this step that outlawed basically all kinds of gloves except for the ones that we felt were the very absolute lowest in latex. It was a very tough step for us to take. It was a tough move just to get the other ones out of the institution. There was a few hundred thousand dollars of new expense that we had to bear because of the . . . situation with latex. The latex was a huge issue that, I think, hit the fan overnight to us, as well as to other hospitals."

Brigham and Women's Hospital was widely recognized for its efforts to control the problems associated with latex allergies. It is somewhat ironic that a hospital dedicated to public health could be the source of life-threatening illnesses. In light of these experiences, the hospital was forced to make a dramatic changes in its healthcare facility. The hospital's decision to implement a multimillion dollar renovation of its existing facility illustrates its commitment to avoiding the problems of the past.

The experiences of the Brigham and Women's Hospital that caused them to convert to powder-free gloves have been a catalyst for other centers to convert to low-allergen, nonpowdered varieties of gloves. The Henry Ford Health System in Detroit elected to switch to powder-free, low-latex examination gloves after determining that the higher cost would be outweighed by savings in Workman's Compensation costs. The Mayo Clinic used a new strategy to purchase surgical gloves. The clinic used Dr. John Yunginger's research data on the allergen protein glove content to select surgical gloves. Since December 1993, Mayo Clinic has used only low-latex allergen gloves. From using 15 to 16 different kinds of gloves before the switchover, the clinic selected only 10 types from five manufacturers. Using the low allergen gloves has actually saved the Mayo Clinic money. Don Scheppmann, director of purchasing for the Mayo Foundation, estimated that, "We are saving $250,000 annually, though this was a byproduct of our effort to get the best product." By standardizing the product of fewer manufacturers, the clinic was able to negotiate for better prices. They also corrected inappropriate uses of the glove. Some surgeons were double-gloving unnecessarily. Other hospital personnel used sterile gloves when they were not needed. Orthopedic surgeons were using unnecessarily costly orthopedic gloves when a regular surgeon's gloves would suffice.

The process of transformation at the Mayo Clinic started approximately three years ago as the head of the Latex Allergy Task Force met on two occasions with the surgical committee to consider glove options. Don Scheppmann explained their strategy to convert to a latex safe environment: "We explained that although they might not be having a problem with latex, a patient might, or another member of their team might. They were quite cooperative." A display was organized of all the low-latex brands under consideration so that surgeons could try on the gloves and ask questions. The surgeons were given an opportunity not to participate in the study. If a surgeon could not find an acceptable glove, he or she could petition for a favorite brand. Of the hundreds of surgeons in the Mayo Clinic, only six have petitioned for a special glove.

The rest of the worker population at the clinic was informed about the planned change through articles in the employee newsletter. Six months later, all gloves with a high level of protein were removed from the inventory. Their stock numbers were deactivated and the unused samples returned to the companies for credit. To help keep glove use under control, Sheppmann monitors all glove acquisitions. The Mayo Clinic continues to monitor glove allergen levels. Recently, a spot check found one glove brand showed a 100-percent increase in latex allergen levels over the year before, and it was pulled from the inventory.

Despite the overwhelming evidence of the dangers of powdered glove lubricants and of high-latex-allergen containing gloves and the frightening experiences of Boston's Brigham and Women's Hospital, many hospitals across the United States persist in a crisis management policy rather than in a proactive stance that protects their patients and employees. Many hospitals continue to use powdered surgical gloves and gloves containing high levels of latex allergens, an invitation to continue the epidemic of life-threatening allergic reaction.

Allergic reaction to latex gloves has now sparked a wave of litigation (Appendix E). Baxter Healthcare (Deerfield, Illinois) has been named as a defendant in approximately two dozen suits according to a report in *Medical Industry Today*. Other defendants include Johnson & Johnson (New Brunswick, New Jersey), Ansell (Eatontown, New Jersey), Becton Dickinson (Franklin Lakes, New Jersey), and Safeskin (San Diego, California). Although the device-makers could not comment on the litigation, Johnson & Johnson spokesperson, Robert Andrews, said that gloves had been used for 20 years and there was nothing better to protect against infectious disease. A spokesperson from Ansell said that the amount of allergy-producing substance in its gloves is the lowest in the industry. The Health Industry Manufacturers Association (HIMA) confirm the claim, saying that glove-makers have reduced the protein levels in gloves and are trying to help hospitals identify people who are allergic to latex.

Plaintiffs are alleging that manufacturers are negligent in failing to reduce protein levels in gloves, unwilling to warn users of possible allergic reactions, and further fraudulently concealing the information about their risk, according to one suit filed by Margaret Williams, a former nurse. Williams, of New Market, Maryland, and others, seek monetary damages. She has alleged in her suit filed in Baltimore's Federal Court that her hands became irritated, her eyes got puffy, and she started wheezing while wearing the gloves during the mid 1980s. She said she was forced to give up her career last year and must continue to avoid products, such as balloons, toys, and erasers. Her lawyer, David Shrager, has three suits pending and could file ten more in the near future. He said that alternatives to the gloves were not marketed as effectively as latex gloves and that his clients had little choice but to use the latex gloves.

The news releases, the television documentary, hospitals' announcements about their efforts to develop a latex-safe envi-

ronment, and litigation involving glove manufacturers all provide strong evidence that the public is now awakening to the
latex-allergy epidemic spreading across our country. Despite this
evidence of increased public awareness, most hospitals continue
to use powdered surgical gloves and gloves that contain high
levels of latex allergens. Until steps are taken by hospitals to set
maximum levels of allowable allergens and prohibit powdered
gloves, the epidemic will continue.

The rationale for the physicians and the hospitals' reluctance
to change to powder-free gloves is based on their naïve perception that the cost of powder-free gloves is an excessive expense
that would interfere with their cost-containment plans in the
competitive managed-care marketplace. When one calculates
the real costs of gloves, one can make these computations from
many different perspectives. If one viewed the cost of one pair of
surgical gloves by a consumer in a pharmacy, one would be
alarmed to find that, in this retail market, the cost of one pair of
powder-free gloves was two- to threefold greater than that of a
glove covered by medicine's deadly dust. However, it is important to emphasize that the purchasing power of the hospital is
quite different from that of the individual consumer. In a whole-
sale marketplace, hospitals purchase literally thousands of surgical gloves so they can effectively barter with the manufacturer
about the glove price. Like the Mayo Clinic, they can successfully use a variety of innovative strategies to lower the purchase
price of surgical gloves.

Another important consideration in calculating the total cost
of powdered surgical gloves is the operative cost to remove the
powder in a sterile manner. After surgeons reported that the cornstarch lubricants on the surface of gloves had numerous adverse
effects on the patient, the FDA in 1971 required that manufacturers place warning labels on the glove packages. The warning label
stated that surgeons should remove the cornstarch from the glove
surfaces by wiping the glove with wet sponges. In a landmark
study conducted by Dr. Margaret Fay, the Global Medical Affairs

Director of Regent Medical Products, and David Dooher, Director of Operating Room Services at St. Luke's Regional Medical Center, Boise, Idaho, the surgical staff's compliance with glove-washing to remove medicine's deadly dust was examined (Table 4.1). The level of compliance among various staff members is illustrated below. The low level of staff compliance with glove-washing is indeed surprising. Only 17 percent of the surgeons washed their gloves after donning. The surgical nursing staff had a slightly higher level of compliance of glove-washing with 21 percent washing their gloved hands. These investigators attributed the slightly higher levels of compliance among nurses to practices taught in nursing school and/or to references to the need for glove washing in nursing journals and textbooks. Information about glove-washing is rarely found in medical textbooks or taught in medical school.

The same study estimated costs associated with washing procedures. Costs were determined by adding basin costs that contained the solution, solution cost, and unit wiping materials

TABLE 4.1 *Staff Compliance With Glove-Washing*

Person	Number (No. Total Personnel Washing Gloves)	Compliance (%)
Surgeons	140 of 827	16.9
Residents	23 of 164	14.0
Interns	0 of 17	0.0
Assistants	103 of 654	15.8
Nurses	164 of 781	21.0
Private scrub nurses	0 of 19	0.0
Technicians	39 of 193	20.2
Circulator-prep	2 of 25	8.0
Physician assistant	0 of 2	0.0
Assistant resident	0 of 4	0.0
Medical student	0 of 3	0.0
Unspecified	2 of 34	5.9

Source: AORN J. 1992; 55: 1500–1519. © 1992, AORN J.

together and dividing by the number of team members. The direct cost of washing materials averaged $0.46 per pair with a range between $0.26 to $1.25 per glove, depending on the materials used and the level of washing required. These findings are disturbing and have serious legal implications for all practitioners who are held to an acceptable standard of practice. Medicine's deadly dust is an increasingly common cause of diseases responsible for serious postoperative complications and morbidity. This study by Dr. Fay and David Dooher provides another strong argument for the use of powder-free gloves.

It is also important for consumers and hospital administrators to realize that some departments in the hospital use powdered surgical gloves in an environment with no easy access to sterile washbasins. For example, emergency physicians in emergency departments treat more than 10 million patients annually with wounds requiring the use of surgical gloves. During their treatment of these wounds, emergency physicians usually do not have the benefit of a surgical nursing assistant to prepare a sterile washbasin filled with saltwater to attempt a removal of the deadly dust from their gloves. Consequently, most emergency physicians use gloves covered by powder during their wound-closure procedures. Few emergency departments have the benefit of powder-free gloves.

When computing the costs of powder-free gloves, another important factor is the durability of the glove or its resistance to puncture. When a glove is punctured, the puncture hole becomes a dangerous avenue for transmission of bacteria and viruses between the physician and the patient. In the same study by Dr. Margaret Fay and David Dooher, it was found that standard powdered gloves were four to seven times more susceptible to puncture than powder-free gloves (Table 4.2). Because the surgeon must change the glove after puncture and don a new pair of gloves, the additional cost of glove replacement becomes another important consideration.

TABLE 4.2 *Failure Rate by Glove Type*

Glove Type	Total Tested	Number of Problems	Failure (%)
White gloves	1,178	106	9.0
Specialty gloves	101	16	15.8
Hypoallergenic gloves	440	54	12.3
Powder-free gloves	1,299	35	2.7
(control)	n = 3,018	n = 211	

Source: AORN J. 1992; SS: 1500–1519. © 1992, AORN J.

Hospital renovations such as that performed at the Brigham and Women's Hospital, necessary to remove the cornstarch from the healthcare facility, must be included in the consideration of the ultimate cost for powdered gloves. The hundreds of thousands of dollars for hospital renovations will be an expense incurred by hospitals in their conversion to a latex-safe environment. Hospitals can, however, justify this substantial expenditure by considering savings in workmen's compensation costs.

As medicine enters an era of managed care, the cost of healthcare has become one of the most important considerations in healthcare delivery. If a new treatment or device could reduce healthcare costs, hospital administrators would welcome it with open arms. Because medicine's deadly dust on surgical gloves is a well-documented cause of intestinal adhesions, it could be strongly argued that surgeons should wear only powder-free gloves in an effort to reduce the incidence of adhesion formation. Conversion to powder-free gloves should reduce the frequency of patients treated for surgical division of adhesions (adhesiolysis) and thereby decrease healthcare costs. The economic impact of hospitalizations for adhesiolysis in the United States is staggering. In a report by Nancy Fox Ray, the cost of hospitalizations and surgeries for adhesiolysis in the United States was studied by pooling data from the National Hospital Discharge Survey, the Medicare Provider Analysis and Review File, and the Part B Medicare Annual Data Beneficiary File. Adhesiolysis was performed during 281,982 hospitalizations associated with 948,727 days of in-patient hospital care. An estimated $1.1799 billion in expenditures was associated with these admissions. Surgeons' fees represented $254.9 million of this figure, while $925.0 million were attributed to hospital costs. Outpatient costs and indirect costs were not estimated in this report. When one considers the billion-dollar price tag for patients undergoing adhesiolysis, the real cost of powder-free gloves is a bargain.

Because a wide range of powder-free surgical gloves is available with low latex-allergen content as well as powder-free, nonlatex gloves, the public is now aware that hospitals can make a latex-safe environment for their patients and employees and end the latex-allergy epidemic. With uncompromised leadership, physicians and administrators should band together to solve this problem in all hospitals in the United States. With increasing public awareness, latex-safe environments will become a standard of care in hospitals in our country.

CHAPTER FIVE

Medicine's Deadly Dust on Surgical Gloves

"Since the days of Ambroise Paré, surgeons might well be divided into two classes. Those who believe what they have been told or have read, and those who believe what they see. There is a world of difference in this philosophical distinction."

Dr. Owen H. Wangensteen

Medicine's deadly dust on sterile surgical gloves is used to fill three roles. First, the dust functions as mold release agent on glove formers during latex glove manufacture. Second, the dust is used as a detackifying agent to prevent the latex of the gloves from adhering to itself. Third, the deadly dust facilitates donning for use in medical and surgical procedures.

Surgeons began using rubber gloves in the operating room 100 years ago to protect their hands and the hands of the operating nurse from the harsh antiseptic agents being used in the operating room. While historians often attribute the use of natural rubber latex gloves to William Stewart Halsted of Johns Hopkins Hospital, Baltimore, Maryland, he was only one of a number of surgeons in the United States and Europe to use protective gloves. In Halsted's time, hospitals sterilized gloves in boiling water, which were then donned by surgeons using water as the donning lubricant. Surgeons donned the reusable gloves by pulling them over wet hands. The gloves formed a water-impenetrable barrier over the surgeon and nurse's hands that ultimately resulted in maceration, or serious skin irritation. Consequently, surgeons searched for dry lubricants that would facilitate donning and prevent wet maceration of the hands.

From the turn of the century until the late 1950s, most surgical gloves were marketed as multiple-use products. As dry sterilization came into practice, these gloves were sterilized, compartmentalized by style and thickness, and dispensed by the hospital central supply department. The development of dry sterilization methods for multiple-use surgical gloves catalyzed the change from wet-donning to the use of dust as a mold release agent and a glove-donning lubricant. Until the early 1960s, after being used in the operating room, contaminated gloves were collected, washed, dried, inspected, powdered with a deadly dust, paired, wrapped and packaged, and resterilized in a steam autoclave for reuse in surgery.

Technological innovations in latex glove processing in the mid 1960s allowed rapid expansion of the disposable medical device industry. Since that time, the vast majority of medical examination and sterile surgical gloves produced by the medical device industry is intended for single use. Modern manufacturing of natural rubber latex gloves is now a highly refined science. The manufacture of sterile surgical gloves has developed into a sophisticated, computerized multistep process combining microprocessors, conveyers, vats, and ovens, which produces consistency in the quality of the glove. The glove's deadly dust may be added during two steps of this manufacturing process.

With the development of dry rubber gloves, some form of lubricity was needed to prevent the sides of the glove from sticking to each other and to permit ease of glove-donning. Powder from *Lycopodium clavatum* was the first deadly dust used as a glove lubricant. *Lycopodium clavatum*, a species of club moss belonging to the fern family, provided the spores used as the first fine powder for surgical gloves. During the late 1800s, surgeons recognized that *Lycopodium* produced inflammatory nodules (granuloma) that were remarkably similar to grapelike masses caused by tuberculosis and cancer. In addition, this deadly dust caused intestinal adhesions.

Intestinal adhesions are stringlike bands that extend in all directions throughout the abdominal cavity. These bands may connect intestinal loops of bowel and extend to the abdominal wall. In some cases, the adhesions cover the opening of the fallopian tubes and prevent sperm from contacting the egg, accounting for infertility. The adhesive bands may attach to the female urinary or genital tract and displace their positions, causing persistent pain. On October 8, 1931, Dr. William Antopol, a pathologist in Bayonne Hospital, Bayonne, New Jersey, described how club moss produced disease in several patients. This deadly dust produced nodules in man that simulated the appearance of tuberculosis or cancer. Because of these disturbing complications, surgeons abandoned the use of *Lycpodium* powder in favor of talcum powder.

Talcum powder or talc mineral is a hydrous magnesium silicate with a theoretical formula of $Mg_3Si_4O_{10}(OH_2)$. It is formed of dolomite or quartzose rocks or by physical alteration of ultramafic and mafic rocks. Talcum powder, produced from ground talc mineral, is a white powder lubricant that is easily sterilized and, in the past, was liberally dusted on gloves and hands to aid in donning. Talcum powder, used in surgery, is a foreign material that remains permanently in the body. When deposited in tissue, it causes inflammation that persists. If polarized light is used in microscopic examination of human tissue, the silicate crystals stand out in brilliant illumination as an electric sign in a night sky. Fibers from gauze and cotton behave in a similar manner when brilliant illumination is provided under polarized light. However, talc can be differentiated from these other foreign bodies by its flat, irregular shape.

Soon after its introduction in the 1920s, talcum powder was implicated in the production of a nodule-like inflammatory mass (granuloma) in tissues and adhesion formation in the abdominal cavity. By 1943, the frequency of talcum powder granuloma was reaching epidemic proportions. Dr. William McKee German in the Department of Pathology of the University of Cincinnati, studied 50 consecutive hospital patients who had previous surgeries and who presented with talc-induced granulomas. Of the 50 patients reported, 40 showed granulomas within the abdominal cavity. Every patient with intra-abdominal granulomas had adhesions! Although a close parallel existed between the number of adhesions present and the number of granulomas, Dr. German attributed the adhesions entirely to other factors rather than just the talcum powder.

It remained for Dr. M.G. Seelig of the Department of Pathology of the University of Washington, in 1943, to demonstrate the danger of talcum powder as an adhesion-producing agent. Although mice are notoriously resistant to the production of adhesions, Dr. Seelig produced generalized adhesions quite consistently throughout the abdominal cavities of mice by directly injecting talcum powder. He also used a starch powder that caused no adhesions. His study represented the first reported use of a starch derivative as a surgical glove lubricant.

In 1947, Dr. Edwin Partridge Lehman, Professor and Chairman of the Department of Surgery and Gynecology at the University of Virginia, verified the increasing evidence that talcum powder played a dangerous role in human surgery. When he dusted dry talcum powder over the intestinal surfaces of several healthy dogs, this deadly dust produced massive, dense, uncountable adhesions wherever the talc came into contact with the tissues. Dr. Lehman's important observations confirmed that talc alone caused adhesions; neither tissue damage nor infection was required. Furthermore, he demonstrated that the talcum powder remained permanently in the abdominal cavity; the human body could not absorb it.

Despite these revelations confirming the dangers of talcum powder, the greatest barrier to the abandonment of talcum powder in surgery was the lack of an acceptable replacement to lubricate gloves. While many powders had been evaluated, each clumped unacceptably during surgical use after sterilization in the autoclave, thereby defeating the primary purpose of the powder, that is, to lubricate gloves and hands. Dr. Lehman believed there was another barrier to the replacement of talcum powder. There was a general failure in most hospitals to appreciate fully its dangers. Dr. Lehman noted alarmingly that, "Surgeons do not even take the precaution of washing the powder from their gloves before operating."

In his landmark experimental study, Dr. Lehman identified an absorbable powder, cornstarch, that he proposed as an alternative to talcum powder. This cornstarch powder contained a small amount of magnesium oxide that served to evenly distribute the powder. He chose a specially treated powder with improved lubricating qualities that would not clump after sterilization. In experimental studies, Dr. Lehman found that the animals completely absorbed the powder left in their abdomens and demonstrated no inflammatory reactions. The cornstarch powder produced no adhesions whatsoever! This newly identified powder was taken up by the cells lining the abdomen and broken down like a starch food. The specially treated cornstarch powder represented a considerable advantage over raw starch and other treated starches because its dusting, lubricating, and flow qualities were not ruined by autoclave sterilization.

In 1949, Dr. R.W. Postlethwait of Duke University College of Medicine, studied the visible and microscopic tissue reaction to cornstarch and talcum powder in dogs by placing these powders in almost every part of the body, including the abdominal and chest cavities and within muscles, tendons, joints, and nerves. He demonstrated that inflammatory reactions to talcum powder were regularly produced in all tissues studied. The modified starch powder introduced by Dr. Lehman, when placed in the same tissues using the identical technique, produced little or no reaction. Consequently, medical science conclusively established that this cornstarch was vastly superior to, and less hazardous than, talcum powder. It comes as no surprise that a survey done in 1952 stated that cornstarch powder had replaced talcum powder in the operating rooms of 60 percent to 90 percent of the hospitals across the United States.

When a new therapeutic agent, like cornstarch, is developed, the tendency is to lose sight of its limitations. While medicine had eliminated the hazard of the deadly dust, talc, Dr. C. Marshall Lee at the University of Cincinnati College of Medicine believed that it was easy to fall into a trap and throw caution to the wind. Dr. Lee stated that, "A widespread impression seems to have developed that starch powder is perfectly safe. There has been a tendency to discard entirely the scrupulous effort to minimize powder contamination of the operative field, which was encouraged when talcum powder was in general use."

Appreciating this dangerous trend, he initiated an experimental reappraisal of the effects of this new absorbable surgical glove lubricant. Dr. Lee ominously implicated this new absorbable powder as another deadly dust. He concluded that cornstarch produced an inflammatory reaction as long as it was present in the tissue. Several variables influenced the intensity, duration, and reversibility of the foreign body reaction produced by cornstarch. The complete dispersal of the powder into individual granules was essential. When adhesions formed because of cornstarch powder, they resulted from clumps or aggregate deposits that could not be absorbed as rapidly as the individual granules. The longer that absorption was delayed, the greater the likelihood that the inflammatory reaction would be irreversible and that adhesions would be permanent. Dr. Lee further discovered that, if infection developed, the resultant inflammatory reaction was much more violent and that permanent adhesions followed. In the absence of infection, fine, individual granules of cornstarch appeared entirely harmless to the abdominal cavity.

In 1952, Dr, Lehman reevaluated the effect of cornstarch in a group of dogs by observing its effect on the abdominal cavity at multiple time intervals instead of only after an extended, fixed period of time as he first reported. He found that, although the starch powder was absorbable, it did produce an inflammatory reaction for the duration of its presence in a wound. Moreover, if clumps of aggregate particles were present, the reaction would be sustained. Concerned about the dangers of cornstarch, he recommended washing the cornstarch from gloves prior to surgery to minimize this danger.

Dr. Lee's concern about the potentially dangerous effects of cornstarch has been verified by literally hundreds of experimental and clinical studies conducted during the last 40 years. Regardless of the site of exposure, scientists documented that cornstarch is a deadly dust that causes serious illnesses that may even lead to death. An enormous body of scientific literature now demonstrates that cornstarch produces a wide variety of tissue reactions. In the abdominal cavity, cornstarch can produce an inflammatory nodule called a granuloma, a life-threatening inflammatory reaction of the lining of the abdominal cavity (peritonitis) and bandlike adhesions.

In 1960, Dr. Richard N. Myers in Philadelphia identified a new clinical entity called starch peritonitis in three patients. These patients had major abdominal operative procedures, from which all three recovered. From 23 days to 25 days after operation, each developed abdominal pain, tenderness, distention, fever, and fluid collection in the abdominal cavity. The three patients were reexplored and the presumptive peritonitis was suspected and later confirmed by biopsy. Dr. Myers replicated this syndrome in experimental trials with healthy female rabbits by spreading varying amounts of starch powder as evenly as possible over the small and large bowel and the parietal peritoneum during laparotomies. Following his clinical and experimental studies, he took definitive steps to prevent this troublesome complication. Before surgery, he rinsed his gloved hands thoroughly in sterile water before each operation. In the

18 months intervening between his last reported case and the time of publication of his findings, he had no additional patients with this starch-induced granulomatous peritonitis.

Over the 20 years that followed the Myers report, numerous reports of starch-induced peritonitis and intraperitoneal granulomas were published in the scientific literature in the United States, United Kingdom, Europe, South Africa, Israel, Japan, and Australia. These clinical reports included studies involved with one patient up to a series of 20 patients. The diagnosis of this starch-induced inflammatory condition can be confirmed by a microscopic examination of one of the granulomatous nodules. With polarized light, the frozen section technique reveals the typical Maltese-cross pattern of cornstarch (Figure 5.1). If the diagnosis was considered after surgery, the surgeon can insert a needle into the abdominal and withdraw a sample of the yellowish colored fluid. Microscopic examination of this fluid would reveal starch granules by iodine staining or polarized light microscopy, providing a rapid, simple means of confirming the diagnosis of a starch-induced inflammatory reaction without the need for unnecessary reoperation.

Starch granulomatous peritonitis is now a well-defined clinical entity. At ten days to four weeks after abdominal surgery, the patient develops abdominal pain, distention, vomiting, and a low-grade fever. The patient's abdomen is usually distended and tender. An X-ray examination of the abdomen reveals distended loops of intestine. The differential diagnosis in these patients usually includes intestinal obstruction caused by adhesions or intra-abdominal infection. Consequently, the majority of these patients have a second abdominal surgical procedure to make the diagnosis. The operative findings include the presence of a large amount of abdominal fluid that may have a yellowish or greenish appearance, grapelike nodules throughout the abdominal cavity, and dense adhesions. These multiple nodules may simulate tuberculosis, or even cancer that has spread throughout the abdominal cavity. While it is accepted that starch

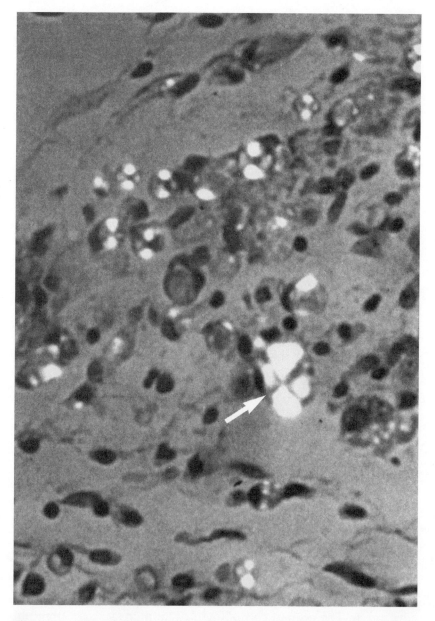

Figure 5.1   This photograph from the microscopic examination of a tissue specimen using polarized light identifies the Maltese-cross pattern for a cornstarch particle (arrow).

granulomatous peritonitis has been elicited by cornstarch on surgeons' gloves, drains, or catheters at the time of laparotomy, there have also been reports of granulomatous peritonitis induced by powder residues placed into the vagina.

The magnitude of the inflammatory reaction in granulomatous peritonitis may also be a reflection of the host's sensitivity to starch. Several investigators have related the inflammatory responses to cornstarch glove powder in patients to immune mediated allergic responses. In 1965, Dr. Barbara Bates in the Department of Internal Medicine, University of Kentucky College of Medicine, described a patient with granulomatous peritonitis secondary to cornstarch following an elective removal of the gallbladder because of chronic inflammation. Cornstarch-induced granulomatous peritonitis was diagnosed at reexploration approximately one month after gallbladder removal. Later, Dr. Bates demonstrated a positive skin reaction eight days after an intradermal injection of cornstarch. No visibly detectable reaction appeared in the control subject. The intradermal injection of the glove supernatant was also associated with an exacerbation of her abdominal symptoms, including steady, generalized abdominal pain, some cramping and distention, and appearance of a single hive. The patient noted onset of the exacerbated abdominal symptoms two days after the intradermal injection.

In 1973, S.T. Holgate from the Department of Surgery, Charing Cross Hospital, England, reported another female patient who developed cornstarch peritonitis one month after gallbladder removal. After questioning the patient, Dr. Holgate found that she had a previous history of skin sensitivity to laundry starch. When Dr. Holgate aspirated fluid from her abdomen, he found many cornstarch particles. After recovery, the patient and six healthy control subjects were given skin injections of cornstarch. The patient complained of an increase in abdominal pain and distention 48 hours later. Dr. Holgate's examination of the forearm revealed a florid inflammatory reaction at both injection sites. The control subjects had no signs or symptoms of allergic reactions to the cornstarch..

Two years later, J.B.F. Grant of the Bristol Royal Infirmary, Bristol, England, performed skin tests with cornstarch glove powder on six patients with proved granulomatous cornstarch peritonitis and also on fifteen control subjects. All patients with starch peritonitis developed a reddened reaction at least 5-mm wide between three days and eight days after inoculation. Such a reaction was not encountered in any of the control subjects. This investigator concluded that an immunologic response plays an important role in granulomatous peritonitis.

The role of cornstarch in producing adhesions in the abdominal cavity has been ascertained by a number of experimental studies. In 1973, D. G. Jagelman and Harold Ellis at the Westminster Hospital, London, England, examined the influence of starch on adhesion formation in rats. When they introduced 100 mg of cornstarch into the peritoneal cavity of rats, they found that it was completely absorbed. When this same dose of cornstarch was used in the presence of injury to the lining of the abdominal cavity, adhesions invariably developed. For Harold Ellis, this study had special significance because it was the beginning of his lifelong scientific odyssey to explain the causes and prevention of abdominal adhesions.

In 1977, S.A.R. Cooke of the Department of Surgery, Johannesburg Hospital, South Africa, examined the significance of cornstarch powder contamination as the cause of adhesion formation in the abdominal cavity of 20 patients subjected to a second abdominal surgical procedure. These 20 patients included 12 in whom the second abdominal surgery was performed within 2 years of the original surgery. Cornstarch granulomas were present in 10 of these 12 patients, indicating that granuloma formation in the early months after surgery is a common phenomenon!

In a pilot study in 1994, Dr. R.W. Luijendijk in the Department of Surgery, Rotterdam, The Netherlands, determined that foreign body granulomas were prevalent in patients with a history of abdominal surgery. In the period from July 1991 to October 1992, all 119 patients on whom abdominal surgery was to be performed and who had previously had an abdominal operation, were examined during surgery for the presence and extent of adhesion formation. Adhesions were found to be present in 94 percent of the 119 patients. In 22 percent of the cases, foreign body particles were present in the adhesion biopsies, caused by the suture thread (16 percent), starch powder from the glove (3 percent), or both (3 percent). The relatively low frequency of starch granuloma was explained by Dr. Luijendijk by the resorption of starch particles in the peritoneal cavity.

A wide variety of complications caused by cornstarch have been demonstrated in literally every part of the body. Cornstarch has been reported to cause inflammation (endophthalmalitis) of the eye after cataract surgery and may result in permanent loss of visual acuity. In addition, cornstarch has been reported to cause thickening of the back muscles that obstructed the connecting tube between the kidney and bladder, obstructing urinary flow. After chest surgery, cornstarch has caused a severe inflammatory reaction that produces chest pain and the development of fluid collections in the chest cavity. Aspiration of the chest cavity revealed multiple cornstarch granules. After heart valve replacement, a patient may develop a collection of fluid within the sac surrounding the heart. As the fluid continues to collect, it may compress the heart chambers, markedly reducing heart bloodflow. Surgical drainage of the fluid collection reveals cornstarch particles. Another patient developed tumor-like nodules beneath the gums after extraction of his teeth. Microscopic examination of the tumor revealed cornstarch granules rather than cancer. Patients have developed swelling of their knees, ankles, and hip joints. Biopsy of the joints revealed cornstarch granules. In these cases, there was evidence that the cornstarch entered the joint space during diagnostic or therapeutic procedures.

Two approaches are designed to prevent the adverse effects of powdered surgical glove lubricants (Figure 5.2). The first removes all traces of powder lubricants from the surface of the surgical glove that contacts the patient. This goal of powder removal is a formidable task when one realizes that each pair of gloves are covered by as much as 700 mg of cornstarch powder. Realizing the potential toxicity of cornstarch, manufacturers have prepared warning labels on each glove packet advising physicians to wash off the powder before use in wounds. Unfortunately, this method of powder removal is ineffective. D.G. Jagelman and Harold Ellis of the Westminster Hospital, London, England, reported that washing reduced the number of starch granules, but left significant cornstarch that appeared to aggregate as clumps on the glove. They postulated that the development of clumps of cornstarch would promote a delay in absorption and an enhancement of the foreign-body reaction.

In 1975, S.J.S. Kent of the St. Thomas's Hospital, London, England, described a method of removing cornstarch powder from surgical gloves. He reported that gloves scrubbed while immersed in a bowl of 1-percent cetrimide solution and then rinsed with sterile water greatly reduced the amount of residual cornstarch on the surface of the glove. The reduction was demonstrated by iodine staining and histologic examination of the omentum in experimental animals after laparotomy with cetrimide-washed gloves.

The most effective method of washing the cornstarch from gloves involves a 1-minute cleansing with 10 mL of povidone-iodine followed by a 30-second rinse under sterile water. This technique reduced the median number of starch granules per mm^2 of glove, as seen on microscopic examination, from 2,720 (when no attempt to remove the powder was made) to 0 (when the povidone-iodine method was performed). This technique is time-consuming, costly, and burdensome to the clinical staff. Further, it cannot ensure that all powder particles have been eliminated.

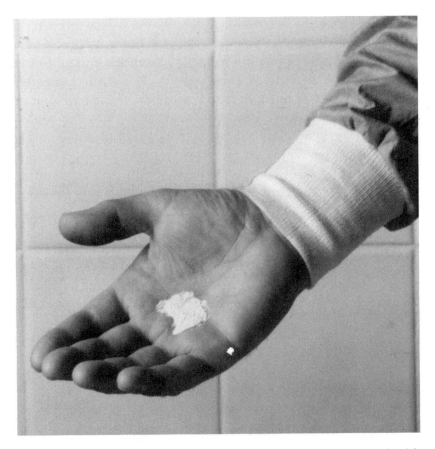

Figure 5.2 The typical pair of powdered latex gloves are covered with approximately 700 mg of cornstarch powder, the amount contained in the palm of this surgeon's hand.

The second approach in preventing the adverse effects of powdered surgical glove lubricants is the development of a powder-free surgical glove (Appendix F). In 1982, a powder-free surgical glove was developed. This powder-free glove is coated with a hydrogel polymer lining that is physically bonded to the natural rubber latex glove and acts as a lubricant to facilitate donning with wet or dry hands. This patented process uses a hydrogel polymer similar to that used in making contact lenses in the United States and has undergone extensive clinical testing for safety. The polymer lining also provides some measure of barrier protection for the wearer against direct skin-to-latex contact. The manufacturing process involves extensive washing and leaching, which is especially important to individuals with sensitivities to latex proteins or accelerators. These polymer-coated gloves are available with a textured or smooth exterior surface. The textured surface of the glove has been specifically designed to enhance the security of grasp of surgical instruments or sutures without diminishing the surgeon's cutaneous sensibility.

The polymer-coated, powder-free surgical gloves are particularly well-suited for tape wound closure. Because the adhesives of wound closure tapes aggressively adhere to the surface of powdered gloves, a physician may have difficulty in manipulating the tape with gloved hands. In contrast, the physician can easily handle skin closure tapes with the polymer-coated gloves because the adhesive of the tape has limited adherence to the glove surface. In addition, the author's investigation demonstrated that cornstarch powder binds aggressively to the tape's adhesive, interfering with the tape's adherence to the patient's skin.

Polymer-coated gloves also have been incorporated into a patented puncture indication system. This double-glove system consists of an inner glove uniformly colored green under an outer glove of neutral color. When the outer glove is punctured, the green inner glove immediately develops a dark patch under the puncture site, a warning to the emergency physician to change the glove immediately. The color change is an optical effect; it does not involve release of dye or any other material but operates on the principle of capillary action. Ingress of fluid causes intimate contact of glove layers, resulting in immediate puncture indication. This double-glove system has two times the resistance to needle puncture as a single glove.

Another strategy in the manufacture of powder-free surgical gloves is surface treatment of the natural rubber latex like chlorination. Natural rubber latex is very reactive toward the halogen elements, acids, and some organic halogen-containing compounds. Chlorinated natural rubber latex gloves are produced by exposing the gloves to chlorine gas or by immersion of one glove surface, or both the inside and outside glove surface, into a solution of the halogen dissolved in water during the final stages of manufacture. This process of chlorination reduces the natural tackiness of the latex. The art in manufacturing these gloves is to balance effectively the slipperiness needed inside the gloves for donning with the grip characteristics needed on the outside surface to handle surgical instruments properly. The ultimate slip properties in the finished glove after chlorination depend on the solution strength, dwell time, and subsequent neutralization cycle. While chlorination improves donning ability and lowers particulate and latex protein levels, it adversely affects the gloves' shelf life, grip, and in-use durability; it may also impart a strong odor. In some individuals, chlorinated gloves have caused skin-irritant reactions. With the advent of powder-free gloves, no justification exists for the continued use of powdered sterile surgical or examination gloves. Given the multiplicity of clinical problems associated with powdered glove usage, physicians will have a difficult time arguing for their continued use.

CHAPTER SIX

Principled Business Leadership in Medicine

"Every innovator has the past to contend with. It is difficult to swim upstream against established opinion."

Dr. Owen H. Wangensteen

In the early 1980s, an American ophthalmologic surgeon discovered a unique solution to the development of a powder-free surgical glove. The idea, however, had to travel all the way to Europe before a powder-free surgical glove could be manufactured and marketed to surgeons in the United States. David Podell, an ophthalmologic surgeon, was one of the first to recognize the potential applications of hydrophilic resins like hydrogel polymers for use as coatings for biomedical devices (Figure 6.1). As a busy ophthalmologist with a successful practice in New York's midtown Manhattan, he had been bothered for years by the seemingly ubiquitous presence of the tiny powder particles from his surgical gloves. These particles frequently attached themselves to his instruments and were often visible during procedures through the oculars of his operating microscope. From his avid reading of medical journals, he was aware of the wealth of medical literature documenting the serious hazards of talc and cornstarch powder glove lubricants in intra-abdominal surgery. He had noted with interest several articles published by ophthalmologic colleagues who reported compli-

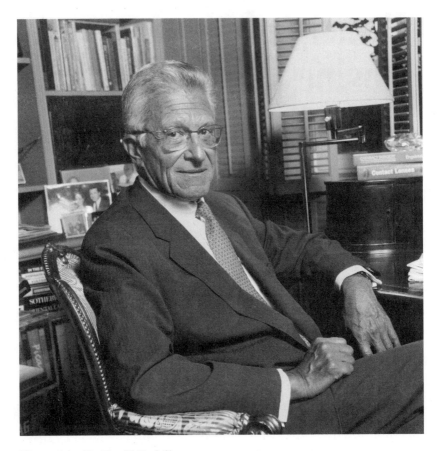

Figure 6.1   Dr. David Podell

cations arising from powdered glove lubricants in their surgical practices. Thus, Podell had long been resolved to carefully wash his sterile gloves after taking them out of their package just before use in surgery. It was not until he experienced a troublesome clinical dilemma in his own practice that he felt impelled to undertake the course of discovery that led to the creation of the first powder-free glove.

Dr. David Podell still vividly recalls when, in 1970, a charming 84-year-old patient experienced a troubling clinical problem as a result of the cornstarch powder coating his surgical gloves.

This elderly Haitian woman had only one eye after losing the other much earlier in life. She came to Dr. David Podell asking for his help in ameliorating new vision problems caused by cataract formation in her eye. He performed the appropriate surgical procedure, intracapsular cataract extraction, without complications. Two days later, however, his patient returned with a severe inflammation of her iris. Her eye looked cloudy and demonstrated a layered level of pus in the anterior chamber, like a half-filled glass of milk. He noted in her chart the diagnosis of early endophthalmitis (inflammation) characterized by recent hypopyon formation (pus level) and anterior vitreous cellularity (cloudiness). Because both bacteria and irritant substances could cause this type of reaction, Dr. Podell considered inserting a needle into her eye to withdraw a sample of the inflammatory exudate to determine definitively the cause of the inflammation, but the risks associated with such diagnostic procedures included the catastrophic loss of the eye. Because of these attendant risks, anterior chamber and vitreous taps were not performed on this elderly one-eyed patient. Also, no attempt was made at intracameral manipulation to recover material from the inflamed eye. Instead, Dr. Podell decided to treat his patient aggressively to cover both an irritant and an infectious cause.

Four days after commencement of this empiric treatment with large doses of intravenous, subconjunctival, and topical antibiotics and steroids, the inflammation cleared to reveal a small cluster of white refractile granules on the face of the iris visualized with his biomicroscope. On recognizing this too familiar sight, that is, the granules of cornstarch powder he saw every day on the surface of his gloves and which literally coated his operating field, his operating needles, his sutures, his surgical instruments, and even his microscope when they frequently fell from his gloves, Dr. Podell knew he had found the source of the problem. He lamented that he could not physically remove the small cluster of starch for fear that this dangerous diagnostic and therapeutic procedure, intracameral manipulation, would put the patient at immediate risk of blindness. Although he was not able to remove and analyze the small cluster of white refractile particles that caused problems for his patient, he attributed the violent inflammation in his patient's eye to the powder-donning lubricant on the gloves used during her cataract extraction operation.

The Haitian woman rarely complained but returned often to Dr. Podell's office to renew prescriptions for the topical corticosteroids she continued to require to control bouts of recurrent inflammation of her iris. Adding insult to injury, she subsequently developed a common complication of topical steroid administration in the eye, steroid-induced glaucoma. This problem required antiglaucoma treatment. Three months after her cataract extraction, the filmy secondary membrane that forms in glaucoma and covered her pupil had reduced her vision to 20/50, and she was still using medicines for her eye on a daily basis. She used the topical corticosteroids and antiglaucoma treatment to control the alternating bouts of inflammation and steroid-induced glaucoma.

Dr. Podell was deeply disturbed by his patient's plight, concerned not only by the ever-returning pus and pain, but also by the decreased vision in her remaining eye. It became clear to him that pharmacologic intervention would offer no panacea in a case such as hers, and that preventing this problem was the only reasonable solution. Feeling strong reluctance to wait still longer for some other individual or group to find the answer that he needed months earlier, he brought his concerns to his cousin, Howard Podell, during one of their customary Saturday morning conferences.

Raised as brothers, he and Howard, a chemical engineer, would meet weekly to discuss their recent collaborative invention, an eyedropper that permitted instillation of ocular medicines one drop at a time in a measured dose. These Saturday morning meetings in the study of David's Park Avenue apartment were times that both men relished. The topic of conversation often strayed down other avenues of thought that ranged from classical music, to education and scientific method, to politics, and to sports. It was a time when David and Howard Podell could bounce innovative ideas off each other, and their conversations often led to practical applications. Howard Podell received his B.S. in chemical engineering from the Columbia University School of Engineering and was a graduate of a three-year training program qualifying him as a registered patent agent. Howard, ten years David's senior, had years of experience as both an engineer and an inventor. He had contributed to the war effort during World War II as an aeronautical engineer in the U.S. Navy, and after the Japanese attack on Pearl Harbor, he was put in charge of converting a General Motors plant in New Jersey to a factory for the production of Navy airplanes. Howard worked as a consulting engineer for General Motors for a time and for his father's company, the Star Fuse Company. He had a special talent for describing complex ideas in simple terms and he used this talent to characterize his many innovative ideas. Thus, he had several patents to his credit. Howard was beloved by his cousin David Podell, especially for his unbridled enthusiasm, his love of discovery, and his ability to take an idea and translate it practically.

David told Howard of his idea to develop a surgical glove coated with a type of plastic polymer in place of the exclusively used powdered glove lubricants. David discussed with Howard a class of hydrophilic resins, called hydrogels, that were used in the manufacture of soft therapeutic and cosmetic contact lenses. Howard was familiar with these hydrogel polymers, which were notable for their slippery surface and their ability to attract and absorb water. David related to Howard the extensive testing undertaken before implementation of the hydrogels in ophthalmology, studies that had previously testified to the safety of hydrogel materials when left in permanent contact with the human body. David felt that this biomaterial would be kind to the surgeon's hands while also safe to the patient. He argued that if the jelly-like hydrogel polymer could be made to adhere to the surface of natural rubber latex gloves, it would obviate the need for the hazardous glove powder.

Howard Podell empathized with David's keen disappoint-ment in his patient's outcome and immediately grasped the potential applications of the hydrogel polymers as a possible substitute for the powder at the root of the problem. In his work as a chemical and mechanical engineering consultant, Howard had developed considerable expertise in polymers and produc-tion-line manufacture. Howard suggested that he and David cre-ate a description and diagram of how the new type of lubricant would be used, which they could use to create a prototype and later use to patent the idea. Their original two sketches and a description of a "... rubber or latex glove of the type used by surgeons which is laminated with an internal plastic lining of hydrophilic material" was submitted to the United States Patent Office. A patent was granted on June 4, 1974, to David and Howard Podell. This patent, number 3,813,695, proposes that the hydrophilic lining could be formed of hydrogels and would serve to reduce "... the friction between the glove and the hand of the user as the glove is applied or removed and eliminates the necessity of conventional lubricating powders such as talc that may contaminate the surgical procedures."

In the weeks following that fateful Saturday meeting, the cousins contacted a well-respected chemical manufacturing company, Hydron Laboratories, which had a history of success-ful marketing of hydrogel polymers. In fact, this company had been instrumental in bringing the technology of hydrogel man-ufacture initially from the Soviet Union to the United States, and Hydron Laboratories held many of the patents for hydrogel applications. Hydron agreed to do a test-coating of one of their patented hydrogel polymers on a sample of commercially avail-able surgical gloves that the Podells washed free of cornstarch lubricant. After polymer application, the resultant pairs of gloves possessed an unworkably thick, leathery coating on their inner surfaces. It was clear that a new, specialized formulation of hydrogels would need to be developed for successful commercialization of the Podells' idea. Hydron Laboratories offered to help proceed with the project development, but the estimate of associated fees submitted by the laboratories seemed exorbitant to the Podells and far surpassed their available working capital.

Undaunted, the Podells contacted a company in Japan that was a major international outlet for the starting blocks used to make hydrogel polymers. The Japanese firm gave them the names of a few chemists in the United States who regularly purchased hydroxyethyl methacrylate (HEMA), a material that was a foundation on which many hydrogel polymers were based. After a few phone calls, the Podells found Dr. Albert Goldstein, a polymer engineer and consulting chemist, educated at Rutgers University (B.S. in Chemistry, 1951) and Cornell University (Ph.D. in Organic Chemistry, 1954), and just the person for whom they were looking. Before forming his own chemical consulting company that specialized in organic chemical manufacture, process and product development, and hydrophilic resins for biomedical applications, Al Goldstein had worked for Hydron Labs for several years as Director of Development. With Howard and Al's knowledge of polymers, and David's knowledge of surgical gloves, they knew they had a team capable of creating a powder-free glove.

Goldstein and Howard Podell set to work in Goldstein's fully-outfitted backyard chemical research laboratory (a cleverly converted one-car garage). In just over a month, they were able to develop an improved prototype of the proposed powder-free glove that demonstrated a level of feasibility far better than the previous prototype. Still, much work remained to develop a marketable powder-free surgical glove.

Howard Podell and Al Goldstein returned to the laboratory. First, they focused their efforts on identifying the appropriate mixture of hydrogel monomers (building blocks) that would combine to form a three-dimensional structure displaying the physical characteristics of a thin, slippery film that would permanently attach itself to the interior of the surgical glove and provide for ease of glove-donning. Next, they spent considerable time and effort delineating the requisite methodology of manufacture, including appropriate solvent for the polymer, treatments of the preparatory glove surface, the method of polymer application, the technique of application, the amount of polymer required, and the necessary cure time and temperature for the polymer that would allow permanent bonding of the hydrogel to the glove.

Their experiments were successful! Other patents followed the first, as the Podells and Al Goldstein perfected the product and the process for making it. The day that Howard appeared in David Podell's office carrying the finished prototypes of the coated surgical gloves and condoms was a memorable one. David found his cousin sitting in the waiting room, flanked by patients on all sides. Howard had his briefcase open in a vain attempt to shield his systematic inflation and deflation of the polymer-coated condoms as he evaluated the polymer lubricant's expansibility and tendency to flake from the latex product. David suppressed his laughter at the sight of his cousin blowing up condoms like balloons amid the raised eyebrows of the two elderly ladies seated nearby. After a brief consultation in the office and a more private demonstration of the merits of this improved prototype, the day blossomed into a celebration for the cousins. The progress made by the ingenuity and perseverance of the threesome seemed remarkable to all of them.

The next step was to find a means to refine the products for assembly-line manufacture and then to bring them to the global market. While they now had the prototype, they did not have sufficient funds to make a commercially available product. David approached several friends and patients, all presidents of their respective corporations based in Manhattan. Many months passed amid a flurry of business meetings where the inventors invariably received the same response: After consultations with research, medical, and marketing advisors, the corporations' management concluded there was no market for a powder-free surgical glove. Venture capital financial support could not be secured because the need for a powder-free surgical glove was not scientifically established in the medical community.

Still undaunted, they approached several American glove manufacturing companies with their plans for the creation of a glove without powdered donning lubricants. The first companies expressed disinterest in the product because there was no perceived market for a powder-free glove. Here too, medical advisors and marketing executives counseled their CEOs that there was no need and no market for a powder-free glove. Several chemists claimed that the Podell-Goldstein glove would not survive manufacture. "It can't be done," they said. "Your glove will curl up like a golf ball," said one.

As often occurs in the tortuous route from fledgling idea to finished product, it was an unusual twist of fate that provided the breakthrough for the Podells and their invention. One late afternoon on a rainy day in downtown Manhattan, Dr. Podell was asked to treat the son of a businessman from England. In his usual custom, he asked the patient's father to tell him about their family and personal lives. When asked about his line of business, the client's father, Alan Woltz, replied, "I make rubbers." Looking out the window at the rain pouring down, Dr. Podell remarked that the rubbers business must be doing well that day. "Not today, but maybe tonight," the gentleman replied. "I make the other kind of rubbers." In the ensuing conversation, David learned that Alan Woltz was a senior executive of a large company in the United Kingdom that manufactured rubber products, including condoms and surgical gloves. David Podell seized the opportunity to tell Woltz of his new collaborative invention and displayed the prototypes for him. Woltz's interest perked considerably. After meeting with Howard and David Podell, Alan Woltz decided to take the prototype to London. A relationship soon developed that led the company, London International Group and its London Rubber Company subsidiary, to strongly consider buying the rights to manufacture the products for the European market.

The Podells asked an entrepreneur, named Howard Miller, to join their team because he was a master negotiator with a disarming use of language that successfully closed deals. Howard Miller also provided a considerable cache of funds from previous business successes that constituted a significant contribution to the development efforts. The Podells, together with Howard Miller, met with Alan Woltz and Michael James, the research and development wizard of London Rubber Company, to discuss how the process had to be adapted to the company's manufacturing process.

Howard Podell and Al Goldstein spent long hours and days in the company's laboratory and manufacturing facility in London, determining how the new process could be matched with the company's equipment and processes to produce a powder-free glove in assembly-line style. First, to eliminate any flaking of the polymer from the inner surface of the glove, it was necessary to maximize bonding of the hydrogel to the latex. Second, the glove had to be manufactured without holes to prevent cross-contamination. Third, the hydrogel coating had to be biocompatible with tissues. The hydrogel was found in these experiments to be safe even if left in tissues and was also found to be nonirritating to the surgeon's hands.

The joint efforts of the Podells, Al Goldstein, and the London Rubber Company's research and development team was a success. After an expenditure of countless man-hours and over an estimated $9 million in premarket research and development, the group had a glove that could be successfully mass-produced. The London Rubber Company and its parent company, the London International Group, negotiated a deal with the Podell group to buy the rights to manufacture the glove and market it in several countries. In 1984, the new powder-free glove was introduced to the market in the United Kingdom under the brand name, Regent Biogel. With a smile, the cousins would tell how the first production-line manufactured glove was as different from Howard and David's initial prototype as the Learjet was from the Wright brothers' Kitty Hawk flyer. The first mass-manufactured gloves donned with marvelous ease when the surgeon's hands were wet or dry, and eliminated the problems of flaking of the polymer from the inner surface of the glove. Within five years of their introduction, the hydrogel-coated gloves had gained 40 percent of the sterile surgical glove market in the United Kingdom, and they were being introduced into other European countries.

Meanwhile in the United States, however, the Biogel glove was not available on the market. When Dr. David Podell requested the London International Group to offer the gloves to surgeons working in American operating rooms, Alan Woltz, Chief Executive Officer of London International Group, agreed to purchase the American patent rights for the product. Alan Woltz sent Nick Hodges, then Vice President of the London International Group, to help secure the deal (Figure 6.2). Nick Hodges and the Podells immediately found a common ground. When Hodges arrived to meet the cousins, he was already a staunch supporter of the Biogel glove. Hodges believed for a long time that the Biogel line should be the core product of his company. Their initial conversations left the Podells not only with a reassuring sense that they had found a new ally, but also with an appreciation for Nick Hodges' seeming genius: his extremely sharp mind, brilliant insight, and tremendous background in the biomedical device industry. The deepest bond was formed by their common dream. "The best part of Nick," David Podell would say, "is his ability to share a vision."

Unlike other executives, the Podells were impressed with Mr. Hodges' work ethics and integrity. These characteristics set him a world apart from his contemporaries. His apparent genius

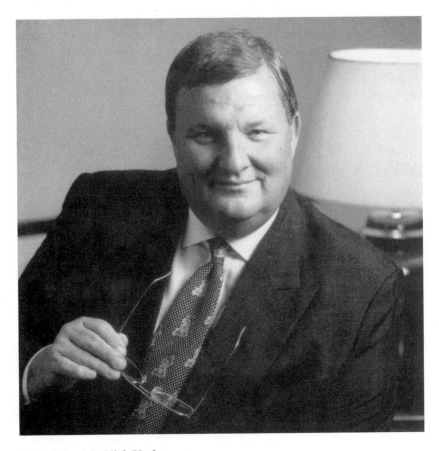

Figure 6.2 Mr. Nick Hodges

lay in his ability to approach this new business challenge in a unique way — combining ethics, science, finance, and marketing know-how, with a complete understanding of the clinical issues surrounding glove powder. His boldness was impressive. His manner conveyed confidence, commitment, and a creative approach to marketing.

Nick Hodges displayed uncompromising leadership. He had serious concerns about the ethics of marketing powder-free gloves and powdered gloves simultaneously because he realized that the cornstarch lubricants were dangerous to patients.

Consequently, he made a responsible ethical decision that had serious financial repercussions. With the support of the Board of Directors, he decided to discontinue the sale of powdered-glove products. This decision cost the company literally hundreds of millions of dollars from hospitals that purchased powdered gloves. He boldly positioned the financial future of his company on the sales of a powder-free glove. His successes in business reflected his uncanny ability to identify leaders in business and science who would join him on this brave adventure to produce the safest glove for surgery. He selected Gareth Clarke to be the Managing Director of Regent Hospital Products, the division of London International Group that manufactured medical gloves. Clarke was an ideal candidate for the position because of his keen sense of business and clear understanding of the science of medical devices. He was instrumental in championing the acquisition of Aladan, Inc., a leading manufacturer of examination gloves. He successfully convinced the employees and managers of Aladan of the merits of manufacturing only powder-free gloves and terminating the manufacture of powdered gloves. He presented eloquent arguments that a powder-free company would become a leader in surgical and examination glove sales in the United States.

While realizing the economic consequences of converting to a powder-free glove company, Nick Hodges, with the aid of Gareth Clarke, charted a new direction for his company that would allow it to assume a leadership role in surgery. He realized that an essential element to his success was his ability to attract a leading clinician and scientist who could direct a multidisciplinary global research program on the performance of surgical gloves.

Dr. Margaret Fay was the ideal candidate for this position because she was a respected clinician and scientist whose research was recognized throughout the world (Figure 6.3). When Nick Hodges offered the position to her, she wanted to be sure that London Rubber was prepared to support a comprehensive, worldwide, multidisciplinary research program. Tempering her excitement with a degree of skepticism, she tried to determine if the firm would commit the necessary research moneys needed to prove causality between powder and patient complications. Knowing the scale of research required to secure an eventual ban on glove powder and the time and cost involved in such an undertaking, she was reluctant to believe that anyone outside the medical community could possibly understand the enormous challenge of such an undertaking. Did they realize that animal studies and clinical trials required to answer causality were expensive? Did they realize the need for a global research laboratory? Were they willing to establish a clinical department?

Even if they made a firm commitment to the program, Dr. Fay realized she would face a dilemma as she moved from animal models to human subjects. No glove manufacturer had ever made a long-term commitment to fund the necessary experiments on a scale large enough to give statistically meaningful results. Yet, Mr. Hodges believed that with properly conducted research, the results would force other manufacturers to think differently about glove products — not as commodity items — but as a medical device. The challenges they would face would be to define rules of scientific conduct that would preserve freedom of academic inquiry, avoid conflict of interest, while at the same time, expedite the transfer of research findings into technologic advancements for their glove products! With little or no objective criteria by which to measure product performance standards, no clinical data to support safety claims for the new powder-free glove, and no guidelines to aid clinicians in objective product selection criteria, Dr. Fay realized she faced a monumental challenge. London International Group would be the first glove company in the world to create a clinical department to sponsor pure academic research in the interest of human health and safety.

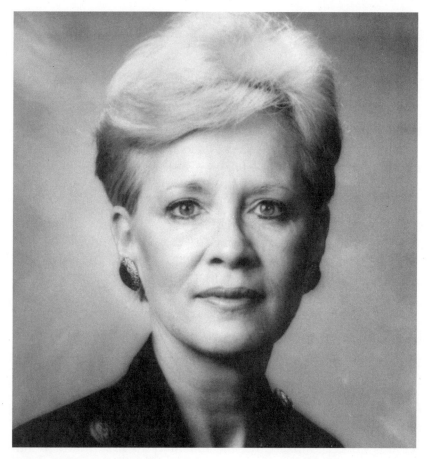

Figure 6.3   Dr. Margaret Fay

For most professionals, motivation comes from enjoying what we do and knowing we are able to make a significant difference in peoples' lives. For Dr. Fay, joining Regent Medical Products meant leaving direct patient care, changing her professional focus, and moving into core research. At the same time, she realized a journey of enlightenment had begun; it was a path that would teach her great humility along the way.

Like many other scientists, Dr. Fay's new "career in science" meant facilitating the research of others, rather than conducting it herself. Frequently, bench scientists and surgeons regard research administrators with considerable suspicion. After all, a facilitator often hinders progress because of commercial interests. Despite these perceptions, Dr. Fay quickly established a solid reputation for advancing research in general and fostering productivity among her scientific collaborators. Realizing the foundation of good biomedical research comes from the bottom up, the real "bench-worker bees," Dr. Fay set out to identify the best scientists in their respective fields.

By the end of 1992, Dr. Fay's core surgical research team proved that the intensity, duration, and reversibility of the foreign body reactions produced by starch granules were greatly influenced by many variables, including the presence of bacteria; tissue trauma inflicted at the time of surgery; particulate debris shed by gauze, drapes, and attire; reactions to suture itself; and poor approximation of the wound. If the team was to prove causality of powder in adhesion formation, however, they needed to advance their studies, moving from cell lines and animal models to actual human subjects.

Scientific accomplishments are much more than the sum of individual efforts. With the full support of Regent management, Dr. Fay conceptualized and implemented the first multinational human study on adhesion formation. World-renowned experts on both sides of the Atlantic included such prominent figures as Professors Dr. Harold Ellis, Dr. J. Jeekel, Dr. Chris Wastell, Dr. Bo Reisberg, Dr. Lena Holmdahl, and Dr. J.J. Duron. For six months, this team labored over a detailed protocol before beginning the project. Taking guidance from Dr. Bill Hartman, Executive Director of the American Society of Pathology Certification Programs, they engineered a method of processing all pathology specimens in Rotterdam to ensure continuity and accuracy of their collective efforts.

The project, which took four years, examined specimens from over 500 patients, all of whom were reoperated for release of adhesions or bowel obstruction. As the research progressed, it became clear that every patient demonstrated some degree of reactivity to powder. Although this group of scientists confirmed causality, that is, powder caused adhesions to form, they noted in some cases that glove powder appeared to cause a hyperimmune response. This observation would be later related to the latex proteins that readily bond to powder.

In 1992, while reviewing Medical Device Reports (MDR) from the U.S. Food and Drug Administration, Dr. Fay discovered a disconcerting trend—allergic and anaphylactic reactions to natural rubber latex gloves. Approaching Regent management, she asked Regent for funds to study "latex allergy." The initial reaction of management was cautious because the firm was considered a leading producer of latex products (gloves and condoms).

The Regent executive team, sharing Dr. Fay's concern for patient safety, took off their "business hats" and put on "scientific hats" to review the data she provided. It was readily apparent that the Regent Hospital products did not cause the same adverse reaction as competitive gloves, but the question was, "Why?" Could it be that the Biogel patented process that allowed them to produce a powder-free glove had somehow removed the majority of allergens from the glove? Clearly, they all recognized a team of allergy-immunology experts was needed to investigate the newly discovered problem. Promoting interactions and cooperation among German, French, British, and American researchers was a daunting proposition. Although the efforts necessary to assemble the team were time-consuming, it was essential to establish a relationship between powder-related complications and allergic reactions to latex.

Building on earlier work in the field of cell reactivity to powder, Dr. Fay returned to the Guthrie Institute where she met with

Drs. William Beck and Donald Beezhold. They were unaware of the burgeoning problem of acquired allergy to latex, chemicals, and some synthetic materials among healthcare workers and patients. Retreating to a boardroom on the main floor of the Institute, Dr. Fay unloaded a ream of case reports showing irritant, allergic, and anaphylactic reactions to natural rubber latex products, antimicrobial soaps, and vinyl gloves. The two distinguished scientists were stunned when they realized the magnitude of the problem.

Although it was known that glove powder would cause irritant reactions in some individuals, until 1979, no systemic allergic reaction to natural rubber latex had ever been recorded. The evidence indicated that nearly 64 percent of all spina bifida patients were affected. More alarming was the fact that between 5 percent and 10 percent of all healthcare workers now showed some evidence of dermatitis, itchy eyes, runny nose and wheezing. Clearly, the problem was allergy-related, but why had it appeared so suddenly? What manufacturing changes had occurred that left high levels of extractable antigens in some products? What were the allergens? Did glove powder play a role in the problem? If it did, could they qualify and quantify the factors leading to the problem?

In the early days of allergy research, it was apparent that Dr. Beezhold would have to create a new assay method that was both sensitive and specific enough to eliminate background artifact. It was this need that led to the creation of the LEAP (latex ELISA for antigenic protein) (Appendix F). Once he created the assay, the team was able to analyze and sequence individual molecular variants of both latex polymers and glove powders. This early research was the first breakthrough in confirming that glove powder was a vector for airborne allergens.

Looking back at that period, one can't believe that Dr. Fay or Dr. Beezhold realized that their work would contribute substantially to an expanded body of knowledge of the biological and immunological reactivity of both glove powder and latex proteins. Neither can one believe that Dr. Fay ever realized the scientific achievements she had accomplished over a six-year period, for they were nothing short of a miracle.

Out of that early work, Dr. Beezhold would emerge from relative obscurity to become an internationally recognized expert in the field of latex allergy. Together with Dr. Gordon Sussman, Dr. Beezhold would proceed to establish a previously unknown key protein in healthcare worker allergy. The two researchers would eventually correlate this protein to cross-reactive reaction to common foods such as banana, avocado, kiwi, passion fruit, potato, and tomato. Dr. Fay created a screening tool for healthcare professionals to serve as a guide in the identification of at-risk individuals. She went on to create the first objective criteria for product selection, thus ensuring that hospital buyers knew the right questions to ask in purchasing safer products.

Because product safety is one of the core principles of her company, Dr. Fay enlisted the support of colleagues at the University of Virginia, Dr. John Thacker, Professor of Mechanical and Aerospace Engineering, and Dr. George Rodeheaver, Research Professor of Plastic Surgery, to study the biomechanical performance of surgical gloves. Because many surgeons believe that powders are necessary to don gloves, especially with wet hands, they are reluctant to change to powder-free gloves. Using a device to measure glove-donning forces, biomechanical studies demonstrated that powder-free gloves are readily donned, even with wet hands. Also, the tactile sensitivity of the surgeon's hands wearing powder-free gloves is comparable to that of powdered gloves. These biomechanical performance tests complement many of the standard tests recommended by the National Fire Protection Association 1999.

For most individuals achieving these kinds of results, it would be enough to rest on their laurels. In the brief span of six years, Dr. Fay had conceptualized, initiated, and facilitated over 212 separate studies, and authored or coauthored over 60 papers. Dr. Fay has always believed that teaching comes from the heart, a gift she has shared with her children. Although she did not set out to transform the world, as the years have passed, she has brought enlightenment to industry, the scientific community, and her colleagues. She was fortunate to find London International Group and its Regent Hospital Products Division, as a place to meet, and work with, an individual like Nick Hodges—a person who shared her vision. Without their dedication and financial support, the answers to the journey she began in 1979 might never have been realized. When asked what she hopes for, she replied, "I hope my headstone will read 'she made a difference.'"

Like a prism held up to the sun, Dr. Fay is filled with innumerable permutations of light, all reflecting a different perception of the world around her. Each reflection casts a new question, opening a new door of scientific discovery. By opening the door to our understanding of factors leading to impaired wound-healing, acquired latex allergy, nosocomial infection, disease progression from adhesions and exposure risk factors from poorly chosen gloves, she has made a difference in all our lives.

On April 22, 1994, Hovey S. Dabney, Rector, University of Virginia, and the Board of Visitors of the University, appointed Dr. Margaret Fay as Research Professor of Plastic Surgery in the School of Medicine. In the Board's appointment letter, Dr. Fay was acknowledged for her exemplary scientific contributions in the area of risk assessment, outcomes research, wound-healing and latex allergy. As she has done since 1993, Dr. Fay continues her collaborative efforts at the University of Virginia in the hope of improving health and outcomes for patients and professionals alike. She has never sought personal recognition for her accomplishments, choosing instead to mentor others in the hope that they will carry the torch of scientific discovery.

CHAPTER SEVEN

Deadly Dusts in Other Medical and Consumer Products

"Cancer has been one of my keen concerns during my tenure here; yet I recognize that we have all been too long on the wrong side of the wood-pile, focusing on surgical treatment rather than prevention."

Dr. Owen H. Wangensteen

In addition to surgical gloves, deadly dusts also coat examination gloves, condoms, and diaphragms. It can also be found on sanitary napkins and in toiletries as well. These powders have caused numerous complications that have had serious life-threatening consequences. They can gain access to the abdominal cavity via two routes: the vagina and surgery.

Substantial evidence exists that material ascends from the vagina to the abdominal cavity (retrograde menstruation). First, surgeons observe menstrual blood in the abdominal cavity when they perform operative procedures on menstruating patients. Second, during surgery and endoscopy of the female reproductive tract, small loose particles of tissue normally lining the uterus have been seen inside the fallopian tubes. Consequently, particles the size of a red blood cell, or even smaller tissue fragments, pass through the fallopian tubes into the abdominal cavity. This retrograde flow of blood and tissue supports the observation that the deadly dusts on surgical gloves, examination gloves, diaphragms, and condoms travel up through the female reproductive tract and gain access to the abdominal cavity.

While the option now exists for the surgical community to convert to powder-free gloves, all currently manufactured condoms harbor deadly dusts. Manufacturers of condoms continue to use a wide variety of dusting powders that include starch, talc, mica, *Lycopodium*, calcium carbonate, silica (silicon dioxide), and magnesium carbonate. In a report in the prestigious journal, *Nature*, in 1988, Drs. Balick and Beitel discovered spores of the club moss, *Lycopodium clavatum*, a potentially hazardous plant product, on a major brand of condom. Dr. Lauri Saxén, a pathologist in Helsinki, Finland, identified cornstarch from condoms when searching for the cause of peritonitis in one of her patients. Unfortunately, condom and glove manufacturers often choose to use particular dusting powders on the basis of its manufacturing characteristics rather than on its potentially harmful effects. The persistent use of these potentially toxic dusting powders on surgical and medical examination gloves is primarily perpetuated by the lack of awareness of the surgeon and the physician about the dangerous effects of the dusting powders. However, recent reports of patients with potentially severe problems, including granuloma and peritonitis caused by starch, occurring in women who had never experienced surgery, may change this uninformed posture.

Deadly dusts, including talc and cornstarch, are also applied to the perineum and genital areas of infants and women. Exposure begins early with baby powders and continues later through the use of body powders, talc for drying the perineum, and cornstarch for the routine maintenance of diaphragms. While the dangerous effects caused by powdered surgical gloves have been extensively documented, dusting powders may also cause illness when used in other situations because of retrograde passage through the female reproductive tract.

Three clinical reports document serious reactions to cornstarch after retrograde passage through the fallopian tubes. In 1957, the British pathologist, Dr. C. G. Paine, documented several patients with abdominal masses due to inflammation ber of small gray or reddish nodules all over the lining of her abdominal cavity. Her pelvis contained the greatest density of nodules, as well as adhesions. Tissue sent for microscopic examination revealed cornstarch-coated particles within the nodules. The patient had no previous surgical history. Dr. Saxén found that the cornstarch originated from the surface of condoms used by the patient and her husband. Dr. Saxén warned that the use of cornstarch-coated condoms may result in infertility.

In 1978, Dr. Denise Hidvegi, a pathologist from Northwestern University in Chicago, provided evidence that douches could induce pelvic and abdominal inflammatory masses because of starch. Her patient, a 59-year-old postmenopausal female, was admitted to the hospital because of vaginal bleeding of two months' duration. The patient had no previous gynecologic or abdominal surgical procedures. Physical examination revealed a nonmobile, moderately firm mass filling the pelvis. During abdominal surgery, her gynecologist found a tissue mass involving the left ovary and firmly adherent to the colon and rectum. Also, countless widespread grapelike tissue masses resembling cancer studded her abdomen. Tissue samples sent to Dr. Hidvegi revealed that the masses thought to be cancer were, in fact, inflammatory tissue containing cornstarch. When her physicians questioned the patient about possible sources of the deadly dust, she admitted to the frequent use of a mixture of water and cornstarch powder as a contraceptive procedure.

Dr. N. Kang and colleagues from the Department of Anatomy in Cambridge, England, conducted the only laboratory experiments to investigate disease caused by condom powders. Powder injections into the abdomen of rats provided a useful method for studying the acute effects of dusting powders. Dr. Kang only tested powders in current or recent use as dusting agents on condoms. All of the tested powders caused harmful effects, including adhesion formation and inflammation within the abdomen, even at the lowest dose. In a 1992 report, Dr. Kang

caused by starch. These patients had had no previous surgeries
The first patient, a 39-year-old woman, sought medical attention
after two days of lower abdominal pain. Her surgeon found a
large, tender, compressible mass arising from the pelvis. She had
no previous surgical procedures and had delivered two norma
babies. A hysterectomy with removal of her ovaries and fallo
pian tubes was performed. Under the microscope, Dr. Paine saw
that the removed tissue contained starch granules in her righ
ovary.

The second patient, a frail 65-year-old woman, complaine
of weight loss and a bearing-down sensation upon walking. He
surgeon detected a painless mass in the right groin. She had ha
no previous abdominal surgical procedures. At operation, he
surgeon found a massive amount of inflamed tissue with tw
masses located in the small intestine and another one in th
colon. Two small nodules from her abdomen were removed an
examined by Dr. Paine, who identified many starch particles i
the biopsy specimens.

The third woman, age 47, worried about her heavy and irre
ular periods for two years. On examination, her physicia
detected masses in her uterus that were judged to be multip
fibroids. She had no previous history of abdominal surgery. He
surgeon performed a hysterectomy with removal of both fall
pian tubes and ovaries. Again, Dr. Paine found granules of th
deadly dust cornstarch in the removed tissue. The pathologi
concluded that, in each of the three women, the deadly dust ha
caused havoc in the abdominal cavity after its introduction in
near the vagina.

In 1963, the Finnish pathologist, Dr. Lauri Saxén, reporte
one of the first cases of starch peritonitis caused by the passa;
of starch from the vagina into the abdominal cavity. The your
woman she described had experienced severe abdominal pai
for two months. Her patient required emergency abdomin
surgery for acute peritonitis. At operation, more than 2 liters
yellowish fluid was removed; the surgeons noted a great nun

ranked the powders based on their relative potential for causing harm, from the most detrimental to the least detrimental: the silicates (including talc), *Lycopodium*, calcium carbonate, magnesium carbonate, and, finally, cornstarch. These findings agree with those of previous studies and indicate that calcium carbonate, magnesium carbonate, or cornstarch should be the dusting powder of choice on today's condoms. In the future, as powder-free gloves replace gloves coated with cornstarch, and the technology improves, powder-free condoms should be developed to replace those using cornstarch.

These deadly dusts can also cause long-term complications in patients. Over the past few decades, talc has been hypothesized to promote the development of ovarian cancer. However, despite extensive research, the theory that talc causes cancer of the ovaries remains highly controversial. Several lines of scientific evidence drive researchers to continue their investigations on the role of talc exposure in the development of malignant ovarian tumors. First, talc and asbestos are structurally similar and commonly found together in mineral deposits. In the past, asbestos fibers have been identified in commercially available talc powder. This natural coexistence of talc and asbestos in mineral deposits raises the likelihood that talc on gloves and condoms may be contaminated with asbestos. Second, asbestos is a known carcinogen with a great potential to induce cancer in certain tissue types. In the tissue lining the lungs and the abdominal cavity, asbestos is implicated in carcinogen-causing mesotheliomas. The tissue of this lung and abdomen lining is very similar to the outermost tissue layer of the ovaries; the two tissue types may be similarly susceptible to cancer. Indeed, in a study performed in 1967, researchers were able to induce ovarian cancers in guinea pigs by exposing them to asbestos. The study also reported similarities between ovarian cancers and mesotheliomas. Finally, not only is talc thought to be sometimes contaminated with asbestos, a substance shown to cause ovarian cancer in some species, but researchers now worry about evidence that the deadly dusts on condoms can ascend from the vagina up through the female reproductive tract to reach the ovaries.

Numerous studies have examined talc exposure in patients with ovarian cancer. These studies have mainly considered talc exposure related to its use as a dusting powder on diaphragms, sanitary napkins, and direct application to the buttocks and genitals. Dr. Daniel Cramer, a gynecologist associated with the Harvard School of Public Health, performed a study in 1982 in which 215 patients with ovarian cancer (and 215 women without ovarian cancer) were assessed for talc exposure by contamination from rubber products, such as condoms, dustings of diaphragms or sanitary napkins, and direct genital application. Dr. Cramer found an increased risk of ovarian cancer in patients who used talcum powder for personal hygiene practices. Specifically, women who regularly dusted their genitals with talc and used it on sanitary napkins had a three-fold greater risk of developing ovarian cancer than women without this exposure to the dusting powder. No increased risk related to condom use or the frequency of abdominal or pelvic surgery was noted. However, Dr. Cramer did note that condom use was not always associated with talc exposure, and he did not obtain specific details about condom brands.

A more ominous series of studies by Dr. Dan L. Longo of the National Institute of Health (NIH) National Cancer Institute and Dr. W. J. Henderson of the Tenobus Institute for Cancer research associated talc to ovarian cancer. In these studies, talc was observed in a number of ovarian and uterine tumors and in normal ovarian tissue. Drs. Longo and Henderson hypothesized that deodorizing talc powders placed on the genitals or the surfaces of condoms and diaphragms reach the ovaries via ascent through the fallopian tubes. In support of this hypothesis, other studies demonstrated that women who had used deodorizing powders on sanitary napkins, but who had blocked tubes and/or hysterectomies, had ovarian carcinoma less often than women with open tubes.

From the University of Washington in Seattle, Dr. Bernard L. Harlow performed a study in 1989 on women who applied talc to their genitals and had borderline ovarian tumors. Dr. Harlow noted an increased-risk factor of 2.8 for women with such exposure. In agreement with the study by Dr. Daniel Cramer, Dr. Harlow did not note an increased incidence of ovarian cancer in women who regularly dusted their diaphragms with talc. That same year, Dr. Margaret Booth at the Radcliffe Infirmary in Oxford found that women who used talc in the genital area greater than once per week had an increased risk of ovarian cancer. Dr. Harlow again studied the relationship between genital talc exposure and ovarian cancer in 1992. This time he assessed frequency and duration of use of talc in addition to modes of genital talc exposure. This study had two significant findings. First, exposure to talc via dusting powder on sanitary napkins, underwear, diaphragms, or husband's use of condoms did not alter women's risk of ovarian cancer. Second, direct genital application of talc did increase the overall risk of ovarian cancer (by 80 percent) if patients demonstrated exposure greater than 10,000 applications. He concluded that a lifetime pattern of genital talc use resulted in a slightly increased risk of ovarian cancer but that it was not a likely cause for the majority of ovarian cancers.

Although all of these studies seem to link long-term direct genital exposure of talc to increased risk of ovarian cancer, the issue is obscured by a number of studies that fail to clearly illustrate this relationship. In 1983, one study of 197 ovarian cancer patients reported no overall association between talc use and ovarian cancer. Dr. Alice S. Whitemore performed another study in 1988 that found only marginally significant elevation in relative risk for ovarian cancer in patients with a history of regular use of talc on the genital area. She stated that, "While these data do not exonerate talc as an ovarian carcinogen, neither do they provide strong evidence to implicate it." Finally, a recent study in 1993 by Dr. Anastasia Tzonou of 189 cases did not reveal an increased risk of ovarian cancer with genital talc application

TABLE 7.1 *Foreign Material on the Surface of Latex Devices Viewed with Polarization Microscopy*

Latex Device	Lot No.	Distributor	Country	Surface Washings*
Ramses Ultrathin condoms	041393	Schmid Labs	Japan	Talc (+) Starch (+++) *Lycopodium* (++)
RIA lubricated condoms	1502	Summa Trading Company	Malaysia	Talc (+++) Starch (+)
Pleasure Plus condoms	0494283	Reddy Distributors Inc.	Thailand	Talc (+) Starch (+++)
TrojanENZ nonlubricated condoms	14828001	Carter Wallace	Not stated	Talc (+++) Starch (+)
Kimono lubricated condoms	30405	Sagami	Japan	Talc (+++) Starch (+)
Sagami lubricated condoms	21108-1	Sagami	Japan	Talc (++) Starch (+)
Gold Circle Coin condoms	17028	Safetex Corp	United States	Talc (+) Starch (+++)
Lifestyle lubricated condoms	310012700	Ansel Products	United States	Talc (++) Starch (+++)

*+ represents rare to few particles (possibly contaminants): ++, few to numerous particles that could be identified in almost every field examined; and +++, maximum density of particles observed.
Source: *JAMA*. 1995;273(11);847. Copyright 1995, American Medical Association.

although they did note that the frequency of reporting talc use was low. Dr. Tzonou concluded that, although her results did not directly link talc as a cause of ovarian cancer, her results could not rule out the possibility. On the basis of these experimental and clinical studies that indicate a potential carcinogenic effect of talc, it would seem prudent to devise safer dusting powders for direct application to the genital regions.

Although talc is no longer used as a surgical glove-donning powder, it still lubricates the surface of many condoms manufactured in the United States and abroad (Table 7.1). Some condom manufacturers have replaced talc and *Lycopodium* with more inert lubricants. A few are diligently working to produce powder-free condoms. Surprisingly, the FDA has not addressed the toxicity of talc on the surface of condoms, even though surgical glove manufacturers are now required to refrain from using talc as a donning agent. To eliminate the risk of talc-associated diseases in sexually active women, condom manufacturers must eliminate all talcum powder used in condom manufacture and work to produce powder-free condoms.

CHAPTER EIGHT

Scientific Paradox: Catastrophic Human Problem, Simple Solution

"At the basis of every achievement of consequence is a good idea, its premise critically tested and the validity of the idea established."

Dr. Owen H. Wangensteen

At this point, readers must be perplexed regarding the paradox of this scientific journey. During the last century, scientists repeatedly demonstrated that medicine's deadly dust on surgical gloves caused serious disease requiring hospitalizations costing society literally billions of dollars. Scientific studies also identified a latex allergy epidemic that threatens millions of healthcare workers and patients and pointed to the significant role of powdered glove lubricants in allergy formation. It must be particularly frustrating to readers when they realize that this staggering problem has a simple inexpensive solution: powder-free gloves with low levels of latex allergens.

If the solution is so simple, readers must question why this apparently straightforward conversion to powder-free gloves with low levels of latex allergens has not been implemented. Readers might hypothesize that there are no agreed-upon, reliable test procedures for evaluating the performance of surgical and medical examination gloves. However, they will soon learn that private nonprofit organizations have developed a plethora of methodologies for testing in the areas of performance and protection that are uniformly accepted by manufacturers, health professionals, and governmental regulatory agencies (Appendix G). Because these rigorous, dependable test procedures are available, readers may then wonder if there is disagreement regarding the performance standards by which gloves products are evaluated. Again, they will be surprised to learn that these same private nonprofit agencies have devised performance standards for surgical and medical examination gloves that are universally accepted. In fact, glove-testing has become such an elegant science that nonprofit agencies are willing to provide a prestigious certification label ensuring the customer of glove performance. What then is the explanation for the failure to implement and enforce these standards? Many believe that the U.S. Food and Drug Administration (FDA) has not taken its leadership role in requiring compliance with these standards by the manufacturers and continues to ignore the evidence.

On December 7 and 14, 1995, the author sent letters to the FDA requesting that the FDA ban cornstarch from surgical gloves. Included with my letter were scientific studies presenting data evidencing that cornstarch powdered gloves caused very similar problems to the original talc powdered gloves. Six months later, Carol J. Shirk, Consumer Safety Officer of the FDA, responded to my letter, assuring me that it was extensively investigating my request (Figure 8.1). Once a policy is determined regarding cornstarch powdered gloves, she indicated they will inform me of the outcome of the review.

Because I have not received any further response from the FDA, I assume that my letter has been smothered in the weeds of bureaucracy. While there may be many reasons for the apparent lack of leadership, such as manpower shortage and other budgetary restraints, its mission of protecting the public can be achieved inexpensively by implementing and enforcing the performance standards already devised by respected nonprofit agencies.

DEPARTMENT OF HEALTH & HUMAN SERVICES

Public Health Service

JUN 3 1996

Food and Drug Administration
2098 Gaither Road
Rockville MD 20850

Richard F. Edlich, M.D.
Distinguished Professor of Plastic
 Surgery and Biomedical Engineering
University of Virginia
Health Sciences Center
Department of Plastic Surgery
Box 376
Charlottesville, Virginia 22908

Dear Dr. Edlich:

This responds to your letters of December 7, 1995, to
Mr. George Kroehling, and December 14, 1995, to Ms. Mary Brady.
Both letters requested that the Food and Drug Administration
(FDA) ban cornstarch from surgical gloves, and encourage the use
of powder free gloves. Included with your letters were
scientific studies presenting data evidencing the cornstarch
powdered gloves cause very similar problems to the original talc
powdered gloves.

Your letters and the scientific data were forwarded to our Office
of Device Evaluation (ODE) for review and comment. We are
advised by that office that the data is still being reviewed and
they wish to spend more time extensively investigating your
information. There is also an internal glove working group that
wishes to review the data submitted by you.

Upon completion of this review, a determination will be made on a
policy regarding cornstarch powered gloves. As that policy is
determined, we will advise you of the outcome of the review, and
the subsequent final policy.

If you have any questions or need further assistance contact me
at (301) 594-4595 or FAX (301) 594-4636.

Sincerely yours,

Carol J. Shirk
Consumer Safety Officer
General Surgery Devices Branch
Division of Enforcement I
Office of Compliance
Center for Devices and
    Radiological Health

Figure 8.1 Letter from Carol J. Shirk, Consumer Safety Officer of the Food and Drug Administration, June 3, 1996.

All glove manufacturers seemingly have a common goal of producing glove barriers that protect the health professional and are safe for both health professionals and patients. This goal is achieved by the development of standard tests that evaluate the performance of the glove, designation of performance standards for the manufactured product, certification of the manufactured products that meet these performance standards, and regulation of the manufacturers of gloves. A number of private agencies use these standards for testing.

Organized in 1898, the American Society for Testing and Materials (ASTM) has grown into one of the largest voluntary standards development systems in the world (Appendix G). ASTM is a not-for-profit organization that provides a forum for producers, users, ultimate consumers, and those having a general interest to meet on common ground to write standards for materials, products, systems, and services. From the work of 132 standards-writing committees, ASTM publishes more than 9,500 standards each year. The ASTM headquarters has no technical research or testing facilities. Such work is done voluntarily by the 36,000 technically qualified ASTM members throughout the world. Membership in the society is open to all concerned in the fields in which ASTM is active. ASTM has devised at least nine different standard test methods for evaluating glove products. These tests measure the following rubber properties: strength, abrasion resistance, flexural fatigue, accelerated aging, puncture resistance, glove dimensions, hole detection, and latex protein levels (Appendix H).

The Association for the Advancement of Medical Instrumentation (AAMI), founded in 1967, is a unique alliance of medicine, engineering, nursing, industry, and government professionals united by the common goal of increasing the understanding and beneficial use of medical instrumentation. AAMI's mission is to assist in the development, evaluation, acquisition, use, and maintenance of medical devices and instrumentation. The association fulfills this mission through certification of healthcare technical specialists, publication of technical documents and periodicals, and continuing education conferences. AAMI Standards and Recommended Practices are written in more than 70 documents contained in six reference volumes. Their recommended practices outlined in volume four, *Biological Evaluation of Medical Devices*, identifies standard tests for biologic evaluation of medical devices like gloves.

The National Fire Protection Agency (NFPA) was started in 1896 as a standards-making organization. Over the years, it has witnessed numerous advances in fire protection, due in large measures to NFPA standards. As the fire-fighters' operations expanded into emergency medical operations, the NFPA developed standards for protective clothing in emergency medical care. Their new standard, NFPA 1999, was developed to address protective garments, gloves, and face-wear designed to protect persons providing emergency medical care against exposure to liquid-borne pathogens during emergency medical operations.

NFPA 1999 defines minimum performance for protective clothing as required by the Occupational Safety and Health Administration (OSHA) Final Rule (29 CFR 1910.1030) on *Protective Healthcare Workers from Occupational Exposure to Bloodborne Pathogens*. The Final Rule states: "When there is occupational exposure, the employer shall provide, at no cost to the employee, appropriate personal protective equipment, such as, but not limited to, gloves, gowns, laboratory coats, face shields or masks, eye protection, mouth pieces, resuscitation bags, pocket masks, or other ventilation devices. Personal protective equipment will be considered appropriate only if it does not permit blood or other potential infectious materials to pass through to or reach the employee's work clothes, street clothes, undergarments, skin, eyes, mouth, or other mucous membranes under normal conditions of use and for the duration of time which the protective equipment will be used."

NFPA offers specific performance criteria for emergency medical gloves:

4-2.1 Sample gloves and related hardware shall be free of rough spots, burrs, or sharp edges that could tear the garment or glove material.

4-2.2 Sample gloves shall be tested for water tight integrity and meet the "pass" requirements when tested in accordance with ASTM D 5151 Standard Test Method for Detection of Holes in Medical Gloves.

4-2.3 Sample gloves shall be measured for physical dimensions and shall meet the length and width dimension requirements when tested in accordance with ASTM D 3577 Standard Specification for Rubber Surgical Gloves

4-2.4 Glove materials and seam samples shall exhibit no penetration of Phi-X-174 Bacteriophage for at least one hour when tested as specified in Section 5-4 of this standard.

4-2.5 Glove material samples shall have an ultimate tensile strength elongation of not less than 2000 psi (13.7 Mpa) and a 300 percent modulus of not more than 300 psi (2.07 Mpa) when tested in accordance with ASTM D 412, Standard Test Methods for Rubber Properties in Tension, Method A, Dumbbell Specimens.

4-2.6 Glove material samples shall be tested for ultimate elongation following whole glove immersion in isopropanol and shall have an ultimate elongation of not less than 500 percent when tested as specified in section 5-6 of this standard.

4-2.7 Glove material samples shall be tested for ultimate elongation following heat aging and shall have an ultimate elongation of not less than 500 percent when tested as specified in Section 5-7 of this standard.

4-2.8 Glove material samples shall be tested for puncture resistance and shall have a puncture resistance of not less than 1.0 lb (0.45 kg) when tested in accordance with ASTM F 1342, Standard Test Method for Resistance of Protective Clothing Materials to Puncture.

4-2.9 Sample gloves shall be tested for small parts dexterity, and test times shall be no greater than 106 percent of baseline test measurements when tested in accordance with Section 5-6 of this standard.

While most of their test methods were based on previously published ASTM standard tests, they also devised some new innovative tests. The Section 5-4 Bacteriophage Resistance Test documents the penetration or passage of this small viral-like particle through the glove. In addition, their Section 5-5 Tear Resistance Test records the tear strength of the glove.

Several private testing services are available for the medical device industry. The North American Science Associates, Inc. (NAmSA) provides pyrogen test specifications for surgical gloves. They use the Pyrogen Test T10 in animals. A pyrogen is a foreign substance that can cause elevated body temperatures much like a fever in patients. Because these pyrogens have been found on the surface of surgical gloves, and in glove powder, they must be removed as they cause a fever comparable to that encountered in postoperative surgical infection. In addition, a standard test for endotoxin using the Limulus Amebocyte Lysate Test is available in their laboratory.

The Underwriters Laboratories Inc. (UL) is a not-for-profit organization that offers product safety testing and certification programs to determine that products meet nationally recognized safety standards. UL also offers quality assessment services for facility Registration. The UL mark represents UL's expertise and signifies a trusted and recognized safety certification. Using the NFPA 1992 standards, it tests gloves to determine if they pass the recommended performance standards. The gloves manufactured by Biosafety Systems Inc. and Absolute Quality Leadership meet these standards and are certified by UL. This product certification is conducted annually.

The Safety Equipment Institute (SEI) headquarters in Arlington, Virginia, is a private, nonprofit organization established in 1981 to administer the first nongovernmental, third-party certification programs to test and certify a broad range of safety and protective equipment. Policy decisions are handled by SEI's Board of Directors, which includes representatives from organized labor, users of safety and protective equipment, the insurance industry, and a safety equipment manufacturer. The purpose of SEI's certification program is to assist government agencies along with users and manufacturers of safety equipment in meeting their mutual goals of protecting those who use safety equipment on and off the job in keeping with recognized standards and the current state of the art. SEI contracts out its testing of personal protective equipment to Inchcape Testing Services, NA Inc. that provides a Certified Product List of personal protective equipment.

The FDA has established basic regulatory requirements for patient examination gloves and surgical gloves. The FDA relies on the voluntary standard issued by the ASTM D 3578-91 for patient examination gloves. In addition to this, glove labeling requirements are necessary. For latex gloves, the principal display panel should read, "This product contains natural rubber latex," "Made of natural rubber latex," or an equivalent statement. The FDA believes that it is prudent to inform users of the identity of the glove-donning powder if used. For this reason, each powdered glove should bear a statement such as, "Powdered (or Pre-powdered) with an absorbable dusting powder U.S.P."

The manufacturer must have appropriate labeling for the powdered gloves. The labeling must comply with 21 CFR 81 and must bear adequate information for safe and effective use of the dusting powder. Also, as announced in the Federal Register of May 25, 1971, 36 FR 9475, the labeling for such dusting powder must include the following information: 1) The recommended use of the powder should be stated as a biologically absorbable dusting powder and 2) The labeling must include the following cautionary statement:

Caution: Powder should be removed from the gloves after donning by washing gloves thoroughly with a sterile wet sponge, sterile wet towel, or other effective method.

The FDA has reviewed its 510(k) policy for medical gloves containing labeled claims of hypoallergenicity and is planning to require removal of hypoallergenic claims from gloves. Afterwards, glove manufacturers will have an appropriate period of time to use their existing labeled stock. The FDA determined that the term, "hypoallergenic," does not have a uniform and well-defined meaning among glove manufacturers. In the future, a medical glove may only state in its labeling that the product is "hypoallergenic," is "safer for sensitive skin," or contain other such phrases that imply a significantly less adverse skin reaction after performing a primary skin irritation study and a dermal sensitization study. Firms wishing to make a "hypoallergenic" claim for surgical gloves must also subject their gloves to a human skin sensitization study known as a Modified Draize Evaluation. The Draize Test was developed by an FDA pharmacologist, John Draize. While this test was originally performed on albino rabbits, the new test will involve at least 200 human subjects. Unfortunately the proposed standard does not address the problem of allergies in latex gloves, it only adds to the problem and must be further revised to include latex protein content.

The FDA also has compliance policy guides for manufacturers of gloves. The FDA will collect samples from lots of gloves to perform the test for defects by the water leak method using 1000mL water. Surgeons' gloves whose leakage defect rates exceed 2.5 percent and patient examination gloves whose leakage defect rates exceed 4.0 percent will be deemed unacceptable. In this event, the FDA will require seizure of the product. European standards are more rigid. They provide a higher level of quality with a maximum leakage rate of 1.5 percent for surgeons' gloves and 2.5 percent for examination gloves.

The FDA also requires that finished gloves be evaluated over the following parameters to ensure that all specifications are met:

- Width
- Length
- Pin holes
- Thickness
- Elongation
- Rips or tears
- Tensile strength
- Powder and/or glove lubricant level
- Color, discoloration, and/or embedded debris
- Measurement or indication of manufacturing material residues
- Measurement or indication of proteins or allergens
- Moisture content or dryness level
- Fisheyes, webbing, or folds
- Package integrity
- Bioburden count
- Labeling

On March 9, 1995, FDA provided interim guidance on protein content labeling claims for latex medical gloves. To encourage the development of improved medical glove products that are low in sensitizing protein content, and in the interest of the protection of public health, FDA will consider 510(k) submissions for reduced-protein latex medical gloves. FDA recommends using the ASTM Standard Test Method for the Analysis of Protein in Natural Rubber and Its Products (ASTM D5712) to help ensure uniformity in protein level determination. This test is to be performed on recently manufactured, finished gloves that have undergone accelerated aging per ASTM D3577-91 or D3578-91. The labeling for a medical glove may include the statement, *"This latex glove contains X micrograms or less of total water-extractable protein per gram."* Labeling for medical gloves with a claim for total water-extractable protein content must also bear the following caution statement:

"CAUTION: Safe use of this glove by or on latex sensitized individuals has not been established."

With the exception of the glove leak test, primary skin irritation test, and total water-extractable protein glove content,
the FDA does not designate specific testing procedures or minimum performance standards for surgical gloves and examination gloves. With the demonstrated coordinated success of the
development of the NFPA 1999 standards complemented by
the independent testing and certification programs, it would
seem prudent that the FDA compile a list of standard testing
procedures to evaluate the performance of examination and
surgical gloves. Like the NFPA, the FDA could indicate minimum performance standard that would allow glove certification. The FDA is well aware of the need for greater regulation
of examination and surgical gloves. In an effort to increase the
level of public health protection, the FDA has taken five
actions:

- Increased the regulatory controls placed on patient examination gloves to bring them in line with the existing
  controls for surgical gloves
- Implemented a more effective test method for detecting
  pinholes and revised the FDA enforcement action levels to
  correspond with the new test method
- Increased the sampling and testing of gloves
- Sent a letter to manufacturers advising them of allergenic
  problems with latex devices
- Conducted an International Latex Conference, Baltimore,
  Maryland, USA, November 5-7, 1992.

On the basis of our extensive experience with testing standards and regulation of examination and surgical glove products, we recommend that the FDA implement the following
additional regulatory guidelines for the glove manufacturers:

- Identification of standard performance tests for surgical
  and examination gloves

- Development of minimum performance standards for surgical and examination gloves
- Banning the use of powdered gloves
- Banning the use of gloves with a high content of latex allergen.

If these recommendations were implemented, the epidemic of latex allergic reactions would end and the complications due to medicine's deadly dust would be eliminated.

Obstacles to Scientific Discovery

"In the lively leaven of an atmosphere fostering inquiry, no one was afraid to come forward with a novel idea, no matter how strange or unfamiliar it may have sounded. In the crucible of experiment and with friendly doubting Thomases looking on, the new idea could be given the acid test. The stages of a new idea are multiple. Many are stillborn. But every new suggestion deserves at least a trial of being blown upon in the hope that there may be sparks in the ashes."

Dr. Owen H. Wangensteen

This epilogue may be uncomfortable for those who fantasize that the road to scientific discovery is usually paved by the intellectual support, unconditional love, and admiration of scientific colleagues. This epilogue is included because the scientists, who are personally responsible for major scientific advancements, are often alone in their beliefs and are sometimes castigated by their well-intentioned colleagues. Those who are made uncomfortable by this assault on the tortuous journey of scientific discovery are warned to read no further. These accounts of the obstacles to scientific discovery are so commonplace that they could fill numerous historical textbooks. Included in this chapter are notable examples that exemplify the struggles of passionate, visionary scientists who overcame these obstacles, making revolutionary changes in our healthcare system.

In his historical masterpiece, *The Rise of Surgery*, Owen Wangensteen reminds us of the tragic story of Semmelweis in his valiant efforts to make innovations in obstetrics. Ignacz Philipp Semmelweis (1778-1865) was born in Hungary and educated in Vienna, Austria. Upon graduation from medical school in 1884,

Semmelweis spent two years working in medicine with Josef Skoda who taught him the difference between testimony and evidence and the value of factual data and statistics. In February 1846, Semmelweis became an assistant to Dr. Johann Klein, Chief of Obstetrics at the Vienna Obstetrical School. At that time, mortality from infection after childbirth was typically 10 percent and could be as high as 90 percent to 100 percent during epidemics. One year later, Semmelweis's friend, Jakob Kolletscka, died following a finger-prick that occurred while performing an autopsy in early March 1847. Semmelweis carefully went over every circumstance and facet of the accident as well as every detail of his friend's postmortem report. He believed that the postmortem findings were the same as those dying of infection related to childbirth. A focal point in his innovative research studies was his connection between the infection identified in the postmortem room and development of infection after delivery in the lying-in ward.

With Klein's concurrence, Semmelweis instituted a program of hand-washing that included scrubbing with a brush in soap and warm water, to be followed by a similar wash in chlorine water until the hands became slippery. This hand-washing procedure was associated with a comparable disinfection of all surgical instruments, linen, and dressings that would come in contact with the mother's birth canal. In two years, Semmelweis had reduced the clinical mortality on Klein's ward to 1 percent. Semmelweis was also able to demonstrate the transmission of fatal birth-related infection to pregnant rabbits directly after delivery by introducing pus recovered from the vaginal tract of women dying of infection after childbirth. Sepsis did not occur if chlorinated lime was also introduced into the rabbits's vagina.

Although Semmelweis did not appear to take an active part in contemporary politics, political developments were destined to have an influence on his career. Semmelweis's chief, Johannes Klein, was a conservative Austrian who was unsympathetic to the independence movement spreading through Hungary.

While he was skeptical of the integrity of native Hungarians, Klein was also worried about the increasing autonomy of traditional values and respect for authority. Concerned about the non-Austrian students, Klein limited their number in his clinic to only two. He justified this change on the belief that non-Austrians were less careful in conducting examinations and were potentially dangerous to the native Austrian patients.

Despite the merits of Semmelweis's enormous scientific contribution, Klein recommended Semmelweis's dismissal to the minister of education. The minister of education accepted Klein's recommendation in light of a developing academic atmosphere that was strongly opposed to innovation. The greatly discouraged Semmelweis returned to his native Budapest as a practicing gynecologist. When Klein died in 1856, members of the Vienna faculty recommended Semmelweis's appointment to the chair of obstetrics at the University of Vienna, but the recommendations of the faculty were ignored.

Semmelweis's book, *The Etiology, Concept, and Prophylaxis of Childbed Fever*, was published in 1860 when he was 42 years old. He expected this book to save the lives of thousands of women who delivered babies in the maternity clinics of Europe. The book was ignored and had little impact on contemporary obstetrical practice. Semmelweis was outraged at the callousness of the medical establishment and began publishing open letters in which he denounced several prominent European obstetricians as murderers. By 1865, his public behavior became embarrassing to his associates and family. By now, he turned every conversation to the topic of childbed fever, and he spoke without taking into account those who might overhear him. By July 1865, his life took a dramatic and sinister turn. His irritating behavior eventually caused him to be involuntarily admitted to an insane asylum. When he tried to escape, Semmelweis was severely beaten by guards, secured in a straight jacket, and confined to a darkened cell. He then developed a serious wound infection in the middle of his right hand that eventually became gangrenous, ultimately leading to his death on August 13, 1865. The cause of death was identified as pyemia, blood poisoning. His death by blood poisoning was similar to the childbed fever encountered in his maternity patients. It is a tragic story reflecting intrigue and lack of vision. History does have a way of repeating itself.

Britain boasts a long unrivaled list of surgeons dating back to the 14th century. In the midst of the 19th century, Joseph Lister (1827-1912) was the greatest of them all. He grew up in a Quaker family. Because he was not a member of the Church of England, Lister could not attend Oxford or Cambridge universities. He entered University College in London at 18 years of age. Lister displayed a greater interest in research than in his scientific studies. It was at Glasgow that Lister instituted his famous trials with carbolic acid for bone fractures that penetrated the skin, an accident for which amputation was the accepted treatment. This amputation was associated with a formidable mortality of 40 percent to 60 percent. In March 1865, Lister started his technique of treating wounds by instilling pure carbolic acid. Later, he used lesser concentrations of 10-percent, 5-percent, and 2.5-percent carbolic acid. In 1871, he devised a carbolic acid spray to be used within the operating room because of his belief that the air of the operating room could serve as a significant source of infection. Lister emphasized surgical hand care; he simply dipped his fingers into a 5-percent solution of carbolic acid to which he added a 0.002-percent solution of corrosive sublimate. The hospital mortality of surgical patients undergoing operations not treated with antisepsis was 4.6-percent, while patients who received antiseptic treatment had a mortality of 2.4-percent. Even though his antiseptic practice was being used throughout Europe, London remained disinterested in his antiseptic practices. Secure in his position at the University of Edinborough, he was always surrounded by throngs of 300 to 400 attentive and appreciative students. When Lister came to London, he often lectured to empty seats. Lister seemed to enjoy the opposition that sharpened his scientific investigations.

ent and ability and to encourage men of promise. From the growth and maturation of such men, come the strength and potential power."

As I have highlighted the many life-threatening dangers of medicine's deadly dust and described the epidemic of life-threatening latex allergies, it should become readily apparent that our healthcare system is faced with an easily preventable crisis. Allergic and other disease-induced reactions to medicine's deadly dust have now sparked a wave of litigation. Consequently, if the cost of gloves covered by medicine's deadly dust was adjusted to include patient care costs for treatment of complications, the price of wash basins used ineffectively to remove the powder, hospital renovations undertaken to eliminate the deadly dust, workmen's compensation claims, and malpractice litigations against physicians and the hospitals, one can only conclude that powder-free gloves are one of the best buys in medicine and medicine's deadly dust should be banned from use in humans.

It is noteworthy to identify some of the obstacles that have blocked efforts to solve this easily preventable healthcare crisis. Because physicians are the leaders of our healthcare system, they must assume the major responsibility. Society still accords physicians a semi-divinity status associated with their practice of medicine where patients seldom question the physicians' actions. Because patient care often involves a patient/doctor relationship in which the physician examines, diagnoses, and dispenses all treatments, many doctors solely assume the authority to determine the best course of treatment for their patients. Many market forces, including governmental regulations and third-party payers, have begun to restrict and regulate physician's choices for their patients. In an effort to retain the authority to determine the best course of treatment for their patients, physicians have had to accept new responsibility for accountability, which takes the form of a willingness to subject themselves to the judgment of peers as well as to evaluate their peers. However, physicians still have considerable hesitancy to question the quality of patient care provided by their colleagues.

In addition to this conspiracy of silence in the medical profession, there are several other factors that have contributed to the physicians' inability to solve this catastrophic problem. One of the major obstacles to medical decision-making is the explosion of scientific information that far exceeds the intellectual capacities of any human being. In the 1990s, the opportunities in medicine placed mankind on the threshold of a new era. Revolutionary advances in genetics at the molecular level, originally developed in simple bacteria and their viruses, have produced powerful technologies that make possible the discovery of the causes and cures of most human diseases. Today, there is the prospect of unparalleled progress in the understanding of human diseases at the molecular level and in developing innovative strategies for their prevention and treatment.

This scientific revolution has been compared to other periods of intellectual and creative accomplishments: the periods dominated by Michelangelo and other great artists of the Renaissance; the music of Beethoven, Bach, and Mozart in the 18th century; and the discoveries in theoretical physics in the first half of this century. The prospects are keenly positive; never before has the opportunity been so great. With the advent of this astounding scientific revolution, computerized information systems are still being developed that can facilitate physician decision-making. Most of these computerized information systems are still not advanced enough to assist the physician at the patient's bedside. Even if they were, many physicians are not comfortable enough with computers to access the information. Medicine's deadly dust has gotten lost in the information overload facing the physician.

Society's misinformed perception of medicine's deadly dust as innocuous dusting powders has further contributed to the physicians' disinterest in this healthcare crisis. When a dusting powder is considered by many to be safe enough for a baby's bottom, how could anyone believe that this powder could be life-threatening?

The continued use of powdered gloves with high levels of latex allergens by most physicians has important implications. First, this decision can be interpreted by the FDA that powdered gloves with high levels of latex allergens are safe for both the patient and healthcare workers. Realizing that the vast majority of health professionals use these dangerous products, the FDA appears to be hesitant to make a decision that will change this accepted practice of healthcare. If the FDA were to make this easily justifiable decision to ban the use of powdered gloves with high levels of latex allergens, the FDA may anticipate that physicians will be angered by the FDA's interference with the practice of healthcare and may attempt to reverse this decision.

Only one glove manufacturer has responded to the requests of the healthcare community. Other manufacturers continue to sell powdered gloves with high levels of latex allergens to the purchaser even though researchers have shown the potential dangers. Cost-effectiveness and profit, not patient protection or worker safety, appear to drive their business decisions. Consequently, they leave the decision regarding glove use up to the physician. Their sales of powdered gloves with high levels of latex allergens is economically a wise decision. In contrast, Regent Medical Products has displayed uncompromised leadership by selling only powder-free gloves with low levels of latex allergens to the medical community. This ethical decision has considerably reduced their potential sales of surgical gloves, a decision that must obviously concern investors in this company.

Because of the continued use of gloves with medicine's deadly dust, it now becomes the responsibility of each individual to demand that physicians use powder-free gloves with low levels of latex allergens. Each individual must assume a new responsibility for their own care and question treatment by health professionals who wear powdered gloves or gloves with high levels of latex protein allergens. If the health professional fails to comply with your request, you should consider finding another health professional who is willing to be your partner in healthcare.

When the patient and physician view healthcare to be a partnership, there are many obvious mutual benefits. First, it facilitates intimate communication between the patient and physician, ensuring that they both agree on the entire diagnostic and treatment plan. Second, patients realize that they play an important role in influencing the outcome of care. This patient empowerment is an excellent method to ensure patient cooperation and compliance with their healthcare. Third, the patient is viewed by the physician as an excellent resource of ideas and information and may alter and change the treatment plan. When these healthcare decisions are made by both an informed patient and physician, the quality and outcome of care will be dramatically improved.

My efforts to empower you to assume this new role in healthcare decision-making may be uncomfortable to you for many reasons. First, you may have a misperception of physicians, viewing them as omnipotent, powerful, and faultless in their professional lives. Overwhelmed by these unrealistic beliefs, it may be difficult for you to have the audacity to believe that you have something meaningful to contribute to the physician.

During my frequent discussions with Dr. Wangensteen, he stressed the vital necessity to inform patients and physicians of the life-threatening effects of medicine's deadly dust. In realizing that medicine's deadly dust could not be removed successfully from surgical gloves, Dr. Wangensteen awaited anxiously for the development of powder-free gloves. Being a dynamic advocate for patient empowerment and education, he lamented over the sluggish indifference that many of his patients had toward their own care. Dr. Wangensteen stated, "I long for individuals to awaken from their torpid lethargy to realize that they alone can powerfully influence their illnesses." His comment

Following Lister's time, extensive experimentation in a number of surgical clinics concluded that it was impossible to achieve absolute sterilization of hands. This finding persuaded most surgeons that rubber gloves were necessary for maximal protection of the surgical patient. Despite these clinical observations, few surgeons wore rubber gloves at the turn of the 20th century. To obviate the need for wearing gloves, Dr. John B. Murphy, Professor of Surgery at the Northwestern University Medical School, in 1904, scrubbed his hands with a 5-percent tincture of green soap in running hot water, washed three minutes in alcohol, and then poured on a rubber solution (Guta-percha), allowing it to dry. He prepared the patients's skin in a similar manner after washing it with ether. He admitted that this practice did not provide as much protection for the patient as intact gloves, but maintained that it was equal or superior to gloves which were subject to a high frequency of perforation.

Dr. Robert T. Morris of New York deplored the decadence that he saw in American surgery, blaming it on the adoption of rubber gloves. He lamented in 1907 that, "We put on gloves for a boxing match with the patient's vitality. . . . The use of rubber gloves made it necessary to use such long incisions that we could work by sight . . . long incisions are used for killing bears."

In 1908, Dr. E. Stanmore Bishop, a surgeon from Manchester, England, deplored gloves as well as face masks and felt that such apparel made the surgeon resemble a high priest of surgery. Mindful of the effects of these vestments upon his followers, Bishop said, "Let us not convert our theaters into the semblance of Muhammadan harems or Spanish torture chambers, nor terrify our patients out of what little courage they still possess." Moreover, he said that gloves make the hands sweat, so that if a glove is perforated, the danger to the patient is compounded. He provided helpful suggestions to his surgical colleagues on steps to avoid using a surgical mask: "Quiet breathing is not specially harmful; it is coughing, sneezing, and loud talking that is dangerous." If the surgeon " . . . feels that he is in danger of sneezing, can he not stoop below the table or for the moment leave it?"

By 1916, Dr. Carl E. Black of Jacksonville, Illinois, indicated that, "Most surgeons seemed to have come to the conclusion that the use of rubber gloves is a necessity and that the protection which they afford against infection outweigh all other considerations. . . . Notwithstanding this consideration, however, there are, no doubt, others than myself who have wished their hands might be freed from the limitation of movement and touch which rubber gloves impose." Black furthermore points out that, "It is well known that a number of surgeons with international reputation for satisfactory technique have never used, or have discarded the use of rubber gloves." Many surgeons did not use rubber gloves because they believed they reduced the sensitivity of touch. Carl Black tested this belief by asking three blind girls to read braille with and without rubber gloves. A definite decrease of sensitivity to touch occurred when wearing the gloves. This decreased tactile sensitivity was more marked when the gloves were dry rather than wet. Even though rubber gloves were introduced in the later part of the 19th century, they were not accepted by most surgeons until the 1920s. Many European and British surgeons did not wear surgical masks until the beginning of World War II.

It is sobering to appreciate the dangers of a critical, devaluing academic environment that smothers creativity. Such an environment existed in the German medical community in which Werner Forssmann practiced in 1929. His mentor and department head, Dr. Richard Schneider, denied Forssmann permission to attempt cardiac catheterization on himself or his patients. Dr. Forssmann was so convinced of the safety and value of the procedure early in the summer of 1929 that he resolved to proceed without the sanction of Dr. Schneider. He relates that, after deceiving the surgical nurse into thinking that she would be the subject and thus gaining access to the necessary instruments, he persuaded her into allowing herself to be tied to the operating table, thereby preventing her from interfering with his plans. He anesthetized the skin of his left arm, advanced a catheter into the right atrium of his heart, and then climbed several flights of stairs to the X-ray department to document his achievement of cardiac catheterization.

It may be very enlightening for us to reflect today on the relevance of the words of Liljestrand at the presentation of Dr. Forssmann's Nobel Prize:

> "It must have required firm conviction of the value of the method to induce self-experimentation of the kind carried out by Forssmann. His later disappointment must have been all the more bitter. It is true that the method was adopted in a few places—Prague and Lisbon—but on the whole Forssmann was not given the necessary support. He was, on the contrary, subjected to criticism of such exaggerated severity that it robbed him of any inclination to continue. This criticism was based on an unsubstantiated belief in the danger of the intervention, thus affording proof that, even in our enlightened times, a valuable suggestion may remain unexplained on the grounds of a preconceived opinion. A contributory cause in this instance was presumably that Forssmann was working in the milieu that did not clearly grasp the great value of his idea."

In the early 1960s the search for an ideally biocompatible material by polymer chemists Wichterle and Lim of Czechoslovakia was a long and tortuous journey. Their odyssey fortunately ended in the first synthetic hydrogel polymer and the subsequent development of soft therapeutic and cosmetic contact lenses. Wichterle's goal was to identify material with optimum compatibility toward living tissue. It had to meet the following criteria: (1) absence of extractable materials, (2) stable chemical and biochemical structure, (3) high permeability for oxygen, nutrients, and other water-soluble metabolites, (4) stable shape, and (5) ability to assume physical characteristics similar to that of the surrounding tissue. When Wichterle went before the Ministry of Health Commission in 1952 with his theoretical basic requirements for an ideal biomedical material, it was clear that such a material had not been identified. The challenge for Wichterle would be to develop a substance to meet these criteria in the face of a commission that rejected this proposal as, ". . . idle talk without practical importance."

Wichterle set out to develop a hydrophilic macromolecular structure that would swell upon contact with water and allow permeability for low molecular weight compounds in solution and removal by diffusion of extractable impurities. He sought to create a structure that became loose and flexible when swollen and yet return to its original shape, even after large deformations. He proposed a structure with hydrolytically stable molecular chains interconnected, ". . . by a continuous sequence of strong chemical bonds." In order to identify a compound that would be inert to biologic catalysts, he proposed that these chains were, ". . . not intended to simulate the chains of biocopolymers, but were to be entirely different, especially from peptide and glycide chains."

Wichterle achieved this monumental task in less than one year of dedicated research. Wichterle reflected at the time, "One has to admit that apart from purposeful efforts, some bad luck was also needed to provide such rapid success." In 1954, Wichterle and Lim collaborated to synthesize a hydrophilic gel by the copolymerization of 2-hydroxyethyl methacrylate (HEMA) and ethylenedimethacrylate for biologic applications. They noted that a number of other monomers belonging to the family of hydrophilic resins could be incorporated to modify the biochemical and physical properties of the basic glycol methacrylate gel. Although variations in the synthesis of hydrogel polymers allow countless applications in the biomedical device industry, the original polymer created by Wichterle and Lim remains the most commonly used biomedical hydrogel today. After a number of successful experimental procedures in animals using the unmodified neutral gel, cross-linked HEMA

One of the main difficulties with linking *H. pylori* to gastritis was Warren and Marshall's inability to develop an animal model for the disease. After failing to infect rats, mice, and pigs, Marshall decided to infect himself with *H. pylori* to see if chronic gastritis developed. In July 1984, he drank a pure culture of *H. pylori* (109 organisms). After being asymptomatic for five days, he experienced early morning nausea and vomiting of acid-free gastric juice. The illness spontaneously resolved after 14 days, but culture and histologic diagnosis demonstrated severe acute gastritis with many *H. pylori* organisms present. This experiment allowed Marshall to link epidemic gastritis with hypochlorhydria to *H. pylori*. It is now accepted that the mysterious syndrome reported by many authors was actually the acute illness associated with *H. pylori* infection. The use by Marshall of self-experimentation is reminiscent of the investigations by Forssmann. While infection of primates with *H. pylori* is obviously safer than Marshall's approach, it is doubtful that he had sufficient grant support for these experimental studies.

Early reports of the association between *H. pylori* and peptic ulcer disease were met with extreme skepticism by physicians convinced that psychic stress, cigarette smoking, and hyperacidity were the main causes of peptic ulcer disease. Nevertheless, with the advent of bismuth-based triple therapy and omeprazole-based antibiotic therapy, convincing double-blind trials were completed, causing the National Institutes of Health to recommend antibiotics for *H. pylori*-associated peptic ulcer disease in 1994.

Dr. Owen Wangensteen, who is considered by many as the greatest teacher of surgery in the 20th century, was very sensitive to the challenges of the creative scientist. He said, "Every innovator has the past to contend with. It is difficult to swim upstream against established opinion." He believed that the most important task of a department head is, ". . . to create an atmosphere friendly to learning. This must be his chief responsibility. He must have a willingness to recognize every type of tal-

Frank Quattlebaum commented that a direct method of coronary artery reconstruction using bypass grafts would be the best surgical solution to the problem. He declined to test his hypothesis in further research studies, anticipating that the results of his scientific investigations would be heard by the same unreceptive authorities. During the next four years, teams of surgeons in other medical centers successfully performed his proposed aorto-coronary bypass graft. By 1972, this new operation became the most frequently performed operation in the United States. Thus, a revolutionary scientific opportunity was missed.

It is not surprising that similar obstacles to scientific discovery are evident in today's academic community. The scientific journey of Barry Marshall, the 1995 Albert Lasker Medical Research Award winner, highlights the importance of the scientist's passion for discovery despite the skepticism of his colleagues. Unraveling the puzzle of the pivotal role of bacteria in gastric disease has taken nearly 100 years. The prevailing dogma was that the stomach was sterile and that bacteria could not survive in gastric acid. Despite this perception, articles described gastric spiral bacteria as long ago as 1896. Descriptions of the presence of curved organisms on the surface of gastric mucosa were ignored by academic medicine.

Fourteen years ago, Warren at Royal Perth Hospital in Western Australia first showed Barry Marshall spiral bacteria (*Helicobacter pylori*) in patients with gastritis. These observations were the beginning of an odyssey searching for a new etiologic factor for peptic ulcers. In a study of 100 consecutive patients undergoing endoscopy, Warren and Marshall identified this new bacteria that could be causally linked to gastritis-associated diseases. In another clinical study of patients with gastritis, Marshall found that bismuth cleared *H. pylori*, but the infection relapsed unless metronidazole was added to the regimen. This therapy was the first shown to heal gastritis, although presentation of the data received a cool reception at gastroenterological meetings.

mind. These hydrogel polymers are being used extensively in medicine today. One of the most innovative applications is the use of hydrogel polymers to coat the surfaces of surgical gloves, thereby avoiding the use of toxic dusting powders.

The road to scientific discovery is a circuitous course in which progress can be slowed by limitations in scientific technology, inadequacy in the design and conduct of the scientific experiment, and the courage, conviction, and commitment of the scientist. The emotional element is the most critical factor. Physicians with low self-esteem, who are overwhelmed by the prejudices of their colleagues, are not likely to succeed.

Early scientific research on the surgical treatment of coronary artery disease is an excellent case in point. In the sixties, during the surgical residencies of Drs. Robert Carlson, Frank Quattlebaum and the author, Dr. Richard Edlich, myocardial vessel implants were the most popular surgical treatments for coronary artery disease. In this operation, a vein graft was attached to the aorta and tunneled into the heart muscle to bring a new blood supply for patients who had previously had heart attacks. Evidence of no blood clots within the vein grafts was the only justification for these procedures. This paucity of scientific information did not deter most heart surgeons from performing this procedure on thousands of patients, making extravagant claims for its success.

In 1966, laboratory investigations performed by Drs. Carlson, Quattlbaum, and Edlich indicated that the contracting heart muscle caused blood to flow in and out implants but did not significantly enhance blood flow to the diseased coronary arteries. With considerable enthusiasm and pride, these doctors shared this information with one of the surgical proponents of this procedure. He abruptly dismissed their findings, reminding them that his patients received excellent clinical benefit from the myocardial implants. Overwhelmed and bewildered by this response, they abandoned further research investigations of coronary artery disease. When they reported the results of their studies, polymer, hydrogel polymers were first used in human surgery in 1954 as orbital implants.

The optical purity of this hydrogel polymer quickly gave rise to the idea of using it for the correction of refractive defects. Dr. Dreifus was the first to use a hydrogel polymer intracameral lens in animals. Although his technique was not attempted in humans, it led to a very effective means of testing hydrophilic materials in the anterior chamber of the rabbit's eye.

Wichterle judged that hydrogel polymer would first be applied clinically as contact lenses. However, he was not successful in enlisting the support of specialists to participate in human trials. "They regarded the idea of an optical device made of rubbery material as ridiculous, and moreover, not amenable to conventional technological procedures." Disregarding the advice of the skeptical scientific community, Wichterle and his colleagues pursued their dreams over several years in the development of hydrogel contact lenses. After six years of futile attempts, the Ministry of Health terminated funding for further applied research for the development of hydrogel contact lenses. The lack of financial support did not end Wichterle's research but only changed the setting for his laboratory. He now tackled that problem at home in his kitchen. At the end of 1961, he developed the first contact lenses by polymerization in open rotating molds, a procedure that most scientists believed to be absurd or unrealistic. During the next five months, Wichterle and his wife produced 5,500 contact lenses in their home, which were tested by Dreifus in the Second Eye Clinic of the Charles University in Prague and later by other ophthalmologists. With this development, new economic implications became evident. Special funds were now made available for the development of three fully automated production lines in the applied section of the research center. Two of these production lines supplied lenses for Bausch & Lomb (Rochester, New York). Wichterle's innovative research provides strong evidence that almost monolithic conservative opposition cannot break the will of the determined and prepared mind. These hydrogel polymers are being used extensively in medicine today. One of the most innovative applications is the use of hydrogel polymers to coat the surfaces of surgical gloves, thereby avoiding the use of toxic dusting powders.

The road to scientific discovery is a circuitous course in which progress can be slowed by limitations in scientific technology, inadequacy in the design and conduct of the scientific experiment, and the courage, conviction, and commitment of the scientist. The emotional element is the most critical factor. Physicians with low self-esteem, who are overwhelmed by the prejudices of their colleagues, are not likely to succeed.

Early scientific research on the surgical treatment of coronary artery disease is an excellent case in point. In the sixties, during the surgical residencies of Drs. Robert Carlson, Frank Quattlebaum and the author, Dr. Richard Edlich, myocardial vessel implants were the most popular surgical treatments for coronary artery disease. In this operation, a vein graft was attached to the aorta and tunneled into the heart muscle to bring a new blood supply for patients who had previously had heart attacks. Evidence of no blood clots within the vein grafts was the only justification for these procedures. This paucity of scientific information did not deter most heart surgeons from performing this procedure on thousands of patients, making extravagant claims for its success.

In 1966, laboratory investigations performed by Drs. Carlson, Quattlbaum, and Edlich indicated that the contracting heart muscle caused blood to flow in and out implants but did not significantly enhance blood flow to the diseased coronary arteries. With considerable enthusiasm and pride, these doctors shared this information with one of the surgical proponents of this procedure. He abruptly dismissed their findings, reminding them that his patients received excellent clinical benefit from the myocardial implants. Overwhelmed and bewildered by this response, they abandoned further research investigations of coronary artery disease. When they reported the results of their studies, polymer, hydrogel polymers were first used in human surgery in 1954 as orbital implants.

The optical purity of this hydrogel polymer quickly gave rise to the idea of using it for the correction of refractive defects. Dr. Dreifus was the first to use a hydrogel polymer intracameral lens in animals. Although his technique was not attempted in humans, it led to a very effective means of testing hydrophilic materials in the anterior chamber of the rabbit's eye.

Wichterle judged that hydrogel polymer would first be applied clinically as contact lenses. However, he was not successful in enlisting the support of specialists to participate in human trials. "They regarded the idea of an optical device made of rubbery material as ridiculous, and moreover, not amenable to conventional technological procedures." Disregarding the advice of the skeptical scientific community, Wichterle and his colleagues pursued their dreams over several years in the development of hydrogel contact lenses. After six years of futile attempts, the Ministry of Health terminated funding for further applied research for the development of hydrogel contact lenses. The lack of financial support did not end Wichterle's research but only changed the setting for his laboratory. He now tackled that problem at home in his kitchen. At the end of 1961, he developed the first contact lenses by polymerization in open rotating molds, a procedure that most scientists believed to be absurd or unrealistic. During the next five months, Wichterle and his wife produced 5,500 contact lenses in their home, which were tested by Dreifus in the Second Eye Clinic of the Charles University in Prague and later by other ophthalmologists. With this development, new economic implications became evident. Special funds were now made available for the development of three fully automated production lines in the applied section of the research center. Two of these production lines supplied lenses for Bausch & Lomb (Rochester, New York). Wichterle's innovative research provides strong evidence that almost monolithic conservative opposition cannot break the will of the determined and prepared must challenge us and cause an explosive wake-up call to all of society. With the advent of powder-free gloves, society cannot settle for less, and must demand that the utilization of deadly dust on medical products be forever banned. With the exclusive use of powder-free medical products, we and our children will be protected from the crippling effects of this deadly dust. Join us in our commitment to healthcare and never bow again to this level of mediocrity. I, like Dr. Wangensteen, challenge each of you to make this dream a true reality.

Carpe diem!

References

The following notes include reference sources and background documents relevant to topics discussed in this book. Entries are organized by chapter and arranged alphabetically for ease of reference by the reader.

Introduction

Antopol W. *Lycopodium* granuloma. Its clinical and pathologic significance, together with a note on granuloma produced by talc. *Arch Path*. 1933;16:326-331.

Dennis C. Current procedure in management of obstruction of small intestine. *JAMA*. 1954;154:463-468.

German WM. Dusting powder granulomas following surgery. *Surg Gynecol Obstet*. 1943;76:501-502.

Lee CM Jr., Collins WT, Largen TL. A reappraisal of absorbable glove powder. *Surg Gynecol Obstet*. 1952;95:725-728.

Lee CM, Lehman EP. Experiments with nonirritating glove powder. *Surg Gynecol Obstet*. 1947;84:689-695.

Wangensteen OH. Credo of a surgeon following the academic line. *JAMA*. 1961;177:558-563.

OH Wangensteen. *Intestinal Obstruction: Physiological, Pathological, and Clinical Considerations with Emphasis on Therapy Including Description of Operative Procedures*, 3rd Ed, Springfield, IL: Charles C. Thomas Pub., 1955.

Chapter Three

Axelsson JGK, Johansson SGO, Wrangsjö K. IgE-mediated anaphylactoid reactions to rubber. *Allergy*. 1987;42:46-50.

Beezhold D, Beck WC. Surgical glove powders bind latex antigens. *Arch Surg*. 1992;127:1354-1357.

Bubak ME, Reed CE, Fransway AF, Yunginger JW, Jones RT, Carlson CA, Hunt LW. Allergic reactions to latex among health-care workers. *Mayo Clin Proc*. 1992;67:1075-1079.

Carrillo T, Cuevas M, Munoz T, Hinojosa M, Moneo I. Contact urticaria and rhinitis from latex surgical gloves. *Contact Dermatitis*. 1986;15:69-72.

Kelly KJ, Setlock M, Davis JP. Anaphylactic reactions during general anesthesia among pediatric patients. *MMWR*. 1991;40:437,443.

Moneret-Vautrin DA, Beaudouin E, Widmer S, Mouton C, Kanny G, Prestat F, Kohler C, Feldmann L. Prospective study of risk factors in natural rubber latex hypersensitivity. *Develop Med Child Neurol*. 1993;35:540-548.

NFPA 1999 *Protective Clothing for Emergency Medical Operations*. 1992 ed., Quincy, MA: National Fire Protection Association, 1992.

Task force on allergic reactions to latex: committee report. *J Allergy Clin Immunol*. 1993;92:16-18.

Voelker R. OSHA mandates universal precautions. *AMA News*. Dec. 16, 1992.

Chapter Four

Beezhold DH, Beck WC. Surgical glove powders bind latex antigens. *Arch Surg*. 1992;127:1354-1357.

Fay MF, Dooher DT Surgical gloves: measuring cost and barrier effectiveness. *AORN J*. 1992; 55: 1500-1519.

Jones RT, Scheppmann DL, Heilman DK, Yunginger JW. Prospective study of extractable latex allergen contents of disposable medical gloves. *Ann Allergy*. 1994;73:321-325.

OR Manager Allergy issues complicated buying decisions for gloves. *OR Manager*. 1995;11(6);1-11.

Patterson P. Stronger glove regs proposed. *OR Manager*. 1990; 6:15.

Ray NF, Larsen JW Jr., Stillman RJ, Jacobs RJ. Economic impact of adhesiolysis for lower abdominal adhesiolysis in the United States in 1988. *Surg Gynec Obstet*. 1993;176:271-276.

Saltos R. Five Brigham operating rooms closed due to faulty ventilation. *The Boston Globe*. July 29, 1993.

Sussman GL, Beezhold DH. Allergy to latex rubber. *Ann Intern Med*. 1995;122:43-46.

Swanson MC, Bubak ME, Hunt LW, Yunginger JW, Warner MA, Reed CE. Quantitation of occupational latex aeroallergens in a medical center. *J Allergy Clin Immunol*. 1994;94:445-451.

Tarlo SM, Sussman G, Contala A, Swanson MC. Control of airborne latex by use of powder-free latex gloves. *J Allergy Clin Immunol*. 1994;93:985-989.

WGBH Educational Foundation *"Can buildings make you sick?"* NOVA Show #2217. Dec. 26, 1995.

Yunginger JW, Jones RT, Fransway AF, Kelso JM, Warner MA, Hunt LW. Extractable latex allergens and proteins in disposable medical gloves and other rubber products. *J Allergy Clin Immunol*. 1994;93:836-842.

Chapter Five

Antopol W. *Lycopodium* granuloma. Its clinical and pathologic significance, together with a note on granuloma produced by talc. *Arch Path*. 1933;16:326-331.

Bates B. Granulomatous peritonitis secondary to cornstarch. *Ann Intern Med*. 1965;62:335-347.

Cooke SAR, Hamilton DG. The significance of starch powder contamination in the aetiology of peritoneal adhesions. *Br J Surg*. 1977;64:410-412.

German WM. Dusting powder granulomas following surgery. *Surg Gynecol Obstet*. 1943;76:501-502.

Grant JBF, Davies JD, Espiner HJ, Eltringham WK. Diagnosis of granulomatous strach peritonitis by delayed hypersensitivity skin reactions. *Br J Surg*. 1982;69:197-199.

Holgate ST, Wheeler JH, Bliss BP. Starch peritonitis: an immunological study. *Ann R Coll Surg Engl*. 1973;52:182-188.

Jagelman DG, Ellis H. Starch and intraperitoneal adhesion formation. *Br J Surg*. 1973;60:111-114.

Kent GJS, Burnand KG, Owen D. A method of removing starch powder from surgeons' gloves. *Ann R Coll Surg, Engl*. 1975;57:212-214.

Lee CM Jr., Collins WT, Largen TL. A reappraisal of absorbable glove powder. *Surg Gynecol Obstet*. 1952;95:725-728.

Lee CM, Lehman EP. Experiments with nonirritating glove powder. *Surg Gynecol Obstet*. 1947;84:689-695.

Lehman WB, Wilder JR. Cornstarch granulomatous peritonitis. *J Abd Surg*. 1962;4:77-80.

Luijendijk RW, Wauters CCAP, Voormolen MHJ, Jeekel J. Foreign body material and the formation of intra-abdominal adhesions. *Dutch J Surg*. 1994;14:138-141.

Myers RN, Deaver JM, Brown CE. Granulomatous peritonitis due to starch glove powder. *Ann Surg*. 1960;151:106-112.

Postlethwait RW, Howard HL, Schanher PW. Comparison of tissue reaction to talc and modified starch powder. *Surgery*. 1949;25:22-29.

Seelig MG, Verda DJ, Kidd FH. The talcum powder problem in surgery and its solution. *JAMA*. 1943;123:950-954.

Chapter Six

Beezhold DH, Kostyal DA, Wiseman J. The transfer of protein allergens from latex gloves. *AORN J*. 1994;59:605-613.

Manson TT, Bromberg WG, Thacker JG, McGregor W, Morgan RF, Edlich RF: A new glove puncture detection system. *J Emerg Med*. 1995; 13:357-364.

Pavlovitch LJ, Cox MJ, Rodeheaver GT, Edlich RF. Considerations in the selection of surgical gloves for tape wound closure. *J Emerg Med*. 1995; 13:353-355.

Pavlovitch LJ, Cox MJ, Thacker JG, Edlich RF. Ease of donning of surgical gloves: an important consideration in glove selection. *J Emerg Med*. 1995;13:353-355.

Swanson MC, Bubak ME, Hunt LW, Yunginger JW, Warner MA, Reed CE. Quantification of occupation latex aeroallergens in a medical center. *J Allergy Clin Immunol*. 1994;94:445-451.

VanMeter BH, Aggarwal M, Thacker JG, Edlich RF. A new powder-free glove with a textured surface to improve handling of surgical instruments. *J Emerg Med*. 1995; 13:365-368.

Wichterle O, Lim D. Hydrophilic gels for biological use. *Nature*. 1960;185:117-118.

Yunginger JW, Jones RT, Fransway AF, Kelso JM, Warner MA, Hunt LW. Extractable latex allergens and proteins in disposable medical gloves and other rubber products. *J Allergy Clin Immunol*. 1994;93:836-842.

Chapter Seven

Balick M J, Beitel J M. *Lycopodium* spores found in condom dusting agent. *Nature*. 1988;332:591.

Cramer DW, Welch WR. Scully RE, Wojciechowski CA. Ovarian cancer and talc: a case-control study. *Cancer*. 1982;50:372-376.

Graham J Graham R. Ovarian cancer and asbestos. *Environ Res*. 1967;1:115-128.

Harlow BL, Weiss NS. A case-control study of borderline ovarian tumors: the influence of perineal exposure to talc. *Am J Epidem*. 1989;130:390-394.

Henderson W, Joslin C, Turnbull A, Griffiths K. Talc and carcinoma of the ovary and cervix. *J Obstet Gynecol Br Commonwealth*. 1971;78:266-72.

Hidvegi D, Hidvegi, I Barrett J. Douche-induced pelvic peritoneal starch granuloma. *Obstet. Gynecol*. Suppl., 1978;52:15-18.

Kang N Griffin, D Ellis, H. The pathological effects of glove and condom dusting powder. *J Applied Toxic*. 1992;12:443-449.

Longo D, Young R. Cosmetic talc and ovarian cancer. *Lancet*. 1979;2:349-351.

Paine C G Smith P. Starch granulomata. *J Clin Pathol*. 1957; 10:51-55.

Saxen L Kassinen A Saxen E. Peritoneal foreign-body reaction caused by condom emulsion. *Lancet*. 1963;2:1295-1296.

Epilogue

Bishop ES. Are gloves and masks advisable in modern surgery. *Surg Gynecol Obstet*. 1908;7:250-2.

Black CE. Some experiments with rubber gloves. *Surg Gynecol Obstet*. 1916;22:701-5.

Brewer GE. Some observations on modern surgical techniques, from an analysis from four hundred and twenty-one operative cases at the city hospital. *Med Record.* 1896;53: 433-436.

Carlson RG, Edlich RF, Landé AJ, Bonnabeau RC, Gans H, Lillihei CW. A new concept of the Vineberg operation for myocardial revascularization. *Surgery.* 1969;65:141-7.

Carlson RG, Edlich RF, Subramanian V, Lande AJ, Bonnabeau RJ Jr., Gans H, Lillehei CW. Myocardial revascularization; II: the role of antithrombogenic mechanisms as a determinant of implant patency. *Angiology.* 1969;20:107-12.

Carter KC, Carter BR. *Childbed Fever: A Scientific Biography of Ignaz Semmelweis.* London: Greenwood Press, 1994.

Forssmann W. *Die Sondierung des rechten Herzens.* Klin Wochenscher 1929;8:2085-2087.

Johnson WD, Lepley D. An aggressive surgical approach to coronary disease. *J Thorac Cardiovasc Surg.* 1970;59:128-138.

Liljestrand G. Cardiac catheterization: development of the technique, its contributions to experimental medicine, and its initial applications to man. *Acta Med Scand.* 1975;579: 7-32.

Marshall BG. *Helicobacter pylori:* the etiologic agent for peptic ulcer. *JAMA.* 1995;274:1064-1066.

Mitchell BF, Adam M, Lambert CJ, Sangu V, Shiekh S. Ascending aorta-to-coronary artery saphenous vein bypass grafts. *J Thorac Cardiovasc Surg.* 1970;60:457-68.

Morris RI. The hand of iron in the glove of rubber. *Med Rec.* 1919;30:273-9.

Murphy JB. A method of dispensing with rubber gloves and the adhesive rubber dam. *JAMA.* 1904;42:1765-6.

Semmelweis I. *The Etiology, Concept, and Prophylaxis of Childbed Fever.* Ed. and trans. K. Codell Carter. Madison: University of Wisconsin,1983.

Wangensteen OH. Editorial: the society of university surgeons and the need for a surgical forum. *Surgery.* 1940;8:120-121.

Wangensteen OH. A surgical pilgrimage. *JAMA.* 1968;205:845.

Wangensteen OH. Historical aspects of the management of acute intestinal obstruction. *JAMA*. 1969;65:363.

Wangensteen OH. University selection criteria for future surgical leaders. *Ann Surg*. 1978;188:114-119.

Wangensteen OH, Wangensteen SD. *The Rise of Surgery: From Empiric Craft to Scientific Discipline*. Minneapolis: University of Minn Press, 1978.

Wangensteen, OH, Wangensteen SD, Klinger CF. Pre-Listerian and Post-Listerian antiseptic wound practice and the emergence of asepsis. *Surg Gynecol Obstet*. 1973;137:677-702.

Wichterle O, Lim D. Hydrophilic gels for biological use. *Nature*. 1960;185:117-118.

University of Virginia Plastic Surgery Research Center Directory of Contributors

"With complete dedication and unremitting industry, some of you may come to stand with your work and discoveries before the courts of posterity and eternity."

Dr. Owen H. Wangensteen

Michael R. Abidin, M.D.
Reid B. Adams, M.D.
Monica Aggarwal, B.A.
Helen C. Ahn, M.D.
Linda C. Ahn, M.D.
Robert C. Allen, M.D.
Richard L. Anderson, M.D.
Lee S. Anthony, Ph.D.
Margaret M. Antoine, M.S., O.T.R.
James Apesos, M.D.
Ann S. Baldwin, M.D.
Vatche B. Bardakjian, M.D.
Leslie D. Baruch, O.T.R.
Erich K. Batra, M.D.
Daniel G. Becker, M.D.
Kenneth T. Bellian, M.D.
David J. Bentrem, M.D.
David E. Berman, M.D.

Linda B. Berry, B.S.
Jessica E. Biesecker, M.D.
Timothy J. Bill, M.D.
Robert F. Bond, M.D.
Timothy J. Brennan, M.D., Ph.D.
William J. Bromberg, M.D.
David E. Bruns, M.D.
Carol A. Bryant, M.D.
Leslie Buchanan, B.S.N., E.N.P.
Lois P. Buschbacher, M.D.
Vincent P. Calabrese, M.D.
Robert W. Cantrell, M.D
Annie Chang, M.D.
Dillon E. Chang, M.D.
Norman C. Chen, M.D.
Van T. Chen, M.D.
Cynthia G. Clapp, M.D.
Lawrence Colley, M.D.

Thomas S. Cook, M.D.
Philip H. Cooper, M.D.
Mary Jude Cox, B.A.
Pamela A. Curtis
Pamela V. Cutler, M.D.
Minh-Chau Dang, M.D.
Olumide Danisa, M.D.
David deHoll, Jr., M.D.
David deHoll, Sr., M.D.
Phillip M. Devlin, M.D.
Allen Doctor, M.D.
Subinoy Das
David B. Drake, M.D.
Julie A. Dunlap, M.D.
Elizabeth C. Edlich, B.A.
Rachel C. Edlich, B.A.
Richard F. Edlich, Jr., B.A.
John M. Eggleston, M.D.
Dina Esterowitz, M.D.
Bruce L. Fariss, M.D.
Brent C. Faulkner, M.S.
Margaret F. Fay, R.N., Ph.D.
Philip S. Feldman, M.D.
Brian L. Ferris, M.D.
Bonnie J. Ford, B.A.
Pamela A. Foresman, B.A.
Earlie H. Francis, III, M.D.
David A. Franz, M.D.
Catherine Gabriel, B.A.
Andrew J. L. Gear, B.A.
Pierre Girard, M.D.
Kenneth E. Greer, M.D.
Dieter H. M. Gröeschel, M.D., Ph.D.
Peter C. Haines, M.D.

Christopher L. Hankins, M.D.
John W. Harbison, M.D.
Carol Hartigan, M.D.
David Herold, M.D., Ph.D.
Jessica D. Hesford, B.A.
Harvey N. Himel, M.D.
Martin A. Hoard, M.D., D.D.S.
Jed H. Horowitz, M.D.
Stuart S. Howards, M.D.
Jim C-S. Hwang, M.S.
Judith C. F. Hwang, M.D.
Elise M. Jackson
Jacqueline D. James, B.A.
John A. Jane, M.D.
Joseph J. Jankovic, M.D.
Matthew Jenkins, M.D.
Kendall C. Jones, Jr., M.D.
Timothy R. Jones, M.D.
David M. Kahler, M.D.
David L. Kahn, R.N., Ph.D.
Helen C. Kaulbach, M.D.
John G. Kenney, M.D.
Elisabeth Kübler-Ross, M.D.
Mical J. Kupke, M.D.
Patricia M. Lampkin, Ed.D.
Scott E. Langenburg, M.D.
Morton H. Leonard, M.D.
Lawrence F. Leslie, B.S.
John Lettieri, M.D.
Mario R. Llaneras, M.D.
Susan A. Lombardi, M.D.
Scott D. London, M.D.
Alejandro N. Lopez, M.D.
Mark H. Lorenzoni, B.S.
Craig A. Luce, M.S.

Michael T. Lynch, M.D.
Theodore T. Manson, B.S.
Mara J. Martin
Craig A. Matticks, M.D.
William A. McClelland, M.D.
Lyle McClung, B.A.
Elizabeth E. McGovern, M.S.
Walter McGregor, M.B.A.
Robert E. McLaughlin, M.D.
Eugene J. Messer, D.D.S.
Paul D. Mintz, M.D.
John C. Moghtader, M.D.
Jaclyn S. Monteiro, O.T.R.
Felice P. Moody, M.D.
Raymond F. Morgan, M.D.
Amy Muir, M.D.
Shahriar A. Nabizadeh, M.D.
Jeffrey G. Neal
Nguyen E. Nguyen, M.D.
Larry S. Nichter, M.D.
Geoffrey D. Nochimson, M.D.
Pieter Noordzij, M.D.
Madeline B. O'Connor, R.N., M.A.
Brett R. Oesterling, B.A.
Stewart O'Keefe, B.S.
Richard D. Paley, M.D.
Bruno Papirmeister, Ph.D.
Sun M. Park, M.D.
Lucas J. Pavlovich, M.D.
John A. Persing, M.D.
Caroline D. Pham, M.D.
Son Pham, M.D.
Lawrence H. Phillips, II, M.D.
David Phung, M.D.

Thomas A. E. Platts-Mills, M.D.
David M. Powell, M.D.
Robert S. Pozos, Ph.D.
Thomas Pruzinsky, PhD
James V. Quinn, M.D.
Vincent E. Rampersaud, B.S.
Joan L. Redd, M.D.
Linda D. Rice, PhD
George T. Rodeheaver, Ph.D.
John C. Rowlingson, M.D.
Karen H. Rheuban, M.D.
Bruce C. Schirmer, M.D.
Robert A. Schwab, M.D.
Jeremy Schweitzer, B.S.
Richard E. Shotwell
Frederick R. Sidell, M.D.
Joseph F. Smith, M.D.
Michael D. Spengler, B.S.
Cornelius V. Stamp, M.D.
Doran R. Stark, M.D.
William D. Steers, M.D.
Richard H. Steeves, R.N., Ph.D.
Brendon H. Stiles, B.A.
Jeffrey D. Stuart, M.D.
Sherry T. Sutton, Pharm.D.
Michael Syptak, M.D.
Scott A. Syverud, M.D.
Allen C. Tafel, M.D.
John A. Tafel, M.D.
Anne E. Tanner, B.S.
Rebecca W. Tanner, M.D.
Peyton T. Taylor, M.D.
William A. Terranova, M.D.

John G. Thacker, Ph.D.
Howard L. Thomas, Jr., Ph.D.
Emily S. Tinsley, R.N.
Michael A. Towler, M.D.
Curtis G. Tribble, M.D.
Blake H. VanMeter, M.D.
John M. Urbancic, M.D.
Haydn N. G. Wadley, Ph.D.
Eric E. Walk, M.D.
Vindell Washington, M.D.
Frederick H. Watkins, B.A.
Lawrence R. Watson, R.D.,
   M.S.
Alissa M. Weaver, M.D, Ph.D.
Susan Faber West, P.T.
Jay J. Westwater, M.D.

Julia C. Wheeler, B.S.
Robert P. Wilder, M.D.
Lee A. Williams, B.S.A.
Sterling C. Williamson, M.D.
Carl L. Wise, R.N., M.S.N.
Lorentz E. Wittmers, Jr., M.D.,
   Ph.D.
Julia A. Woods, B.A.
Heather R. Wright, B.A.
Melissa M. Wu, M.D.
Gregory C. Zachmann, M.D.
Neil J. Zemmel, B.S.
Christopher A. Zimmer, M.D
Jesse E. Zook
Marianne Zura, B.A.
Robert D. Zura, M.D.

University of Virginia Plastic Surgery Research Center Directory of Sponsors

"Plant a tree for posterity in the orchard of your profession that will give you enduring satisfaction though you may never live to see it mature; its growth can project your image and wishes far into time and space."

Dr. Owen H. Wangensteen

Edward S. Arnold
Edmund Bingham
Roger E. Birk
Michael Bloomberg
Linda Blumenfeld
Michael L. Blumenfeld, D.D.S.
John P. Brandel
Carr-Scarborough Microbials
Donald Cecil
Charles Edison Fund
John A. Crane
Gerald E. Cremins
Patricia and Edward Davis
Hugh Devlin
Enhance Financial Services Group, Inc.
George Newton Bullard Foundation
George P. Green

Harvey R. Heller
Peter W. Henderson
Kim and Chris Henderson
Daniel A. Hoffler
Virginia E. Holt
Robert M. Howard, Jr.
Ira W. DeCamp Foundation
Jandon Foundation
Charles H. Jones, Jr.
David Jones
Esther and Leonard Kurtz
Loomis C. Leedy, Jr.
John C. McCrane
Nancy Lee and Herbert McKay
Merrill Lynch and Company Foundation
Merril Lynch Asset Management, Inc.

Roger Milliken
William G. Moore
J. Michael Muckleroy
Palmer Weber Research Fund
James Peake
Theodore J. Reiss
Beth and Charles H. Ross, Jr.
Bryan Satterlee
Saunders Foundation
Wallace O. Sellers
Ghassan I. Shaker
Winthrop H. Smith, Jr.
Southern Medical Association
Spectrum Emergency Care,
 Inc.

Ruth E. Tanner
William Tanner
Teco Energy
Texaco Foundation
3M Center
Richard H. Tierney
Lee and J. Thomas Touchton
Trigon Blue Cross-Blue Shield
Daniel P. Tully
U. S. Surgical Corporation
Roger M. Vasey
Alexander J. von Thelen
David Ward
Van Whisnand
James T. Wolfensohn

Technical Factors in the Diagnosis of Latex Allergry

Diagnosis

Diagnosis of latex allergy depends upon the sequential use of serologic, use, and skin-prick tests to optimize safety, diagnostic sensitivity, and specificity. Physicians should offer serologic testing at a reputable laboratory to symptomatic patients with a possible latex allergy. If serologic testing is positive, latex allergy is confirmed, and no further testing is necessary. If serologic testing is negative in a symptomatic patient, a use test should be performed. If the use test is positive, latex allergy is confirmed. If the use test is negative, a skin-prick test is performed as the final diagnostic tool. A negative prick or serologic tests performed shortly after an acute latex response might reflect a "false negative" because an immunologic refractory period similar to that encountered after a bee sting.

Skin-Prick Testing

Of the currently available tests, skin-prick testing is the most reliable. This test has the advantages of being sensitive, rapid, and cost-effective. Reports of anaphylaxis during skin-prick testing for latex allergy emphasize the need for safe testing methods for diagnosis.[1,2] Any skin-prick testing should be done by trained allergists in a hospital setting with adequate resuscitation and medical support services and an intravenous infusion readily available to rapidly provide epinephrine, volume expanders, and vasopressor agents in the event of a reaction. Although available abroad, there is no commercially available, FDA-approved, latex skin extract in the United States. Consequently, American allergists who wish to perform latex skin prick testing should follow experimental protocols.[3] Outside of the United States, commercial nonstandardized extracts have proven effective for skin-prick testing and are considered safe when initial testing is performed with a 10- or 100-fold dilution to yield an extract with a < 1 ng/mL concentration.

In-Vitro Assays for Latex-Specific IgE

Sensitive and specific commercial in-vitro serologic assays that have been developed for the diagnosis of IgE mediated latex allergy include an immunoflouro-assay, Pharmacia CAP (Pharmacia Diagnostics, Inc., Piscataway, New Jersey) and an ELISA assay, AlaSTAT (AlaSTAT Diagnostic Products Corporation, Los Angeles, California).

The differences in latex source materials used in latex exposure and the existence of possible cross-reacting antibodies contribute to variance in the accuracy of these tests. If the latex antigens in the sensitizing product are different from the epitopes used in the assay, a false negative test result may occur. In atopic individuals, especially patients with allergies to fruits and/or vegetables, these serologic tests can produce false positive results. All serological testing for latex allergy should be preferred by experienced laboratories.

Use Test

The "use test" described by Kelly is useful in patients with a compelling history, but with a negative serologic assay. The use test should be preceded by an explanation of the attendant risks and benefits.[4] The use test is performed with a fingertip cut from a sterile surgical glove, moistened with saline, and applied to the skin of the patient for a 15-minute period. Urticarial pruritus or erythema is indicative of a positive result. If no reaction is noted, an entire saline-moistened surgical glove can then be placed on the hand of the patient until a reaction ensues, or for a maximum of 15 minutes. However, patient safety during full glove-use testing is ill-defined, and is dependent on the allergenicity of latex proteins in the surgical glove used for the test.

Patch Testing

Patch testing is helpful in differentiating between irritant contact dermatitis and allergic contact dermatitis mediated by type IV hypersensitivity reactions. The patch test is the definitive test for diagnosis of patients with type IV hypersensitivity to latex products. For patients presenting with only contact dermatitis or urticaria, diagnosis may be facilitated with patch testing using a standard battery of rubber additives. Accelerators evoke positive patch tests in 32 of 39 patients (82 percent) with occupationally induced contact dermatitis associated with glove use.[5]

The allergen is applied on normal skin, usually on the patient's back or arms, under a small semiocclusive dressing. When testing for allergic hypersensitivity, avoid applying test substances in concentrations with the inherent capacity to cause visible changes even on nonsensitized normal skin. The standard screening tray of the North American Contact Dermatitis Group contains a series of common contact allergens, which include those found in surgical gloves and are useful for patch testing; this battery includes p-pheynlenediamine 1 percent, mercaptobenzothiazole 1 percent, mercapto-mix 1 percent, thiuram-mix 1 percent, and carba-mix 3 percent.

Patch tests are left in place for 24 hours to 48 hours. The results are first read about 30 minutes after removal of the patches and again 24 hours or 48 hours later. Before a substance that has elicited a positive reaction can be accepted as the cause of the presenting eruption, the result of each patch test must be associated with the history of allergenic exposures and with clinical findings. It is important to emphasize a risk of inducing contact sensitization by exposures involved in patch tests; however, this risk should not interfere with the judicious use of this form of testing.

Management of Latex Allergies

Management of a latex-allergic patient in an ambulance or the emergency department can be very difficult because latex is ubiquitous in medical environments. Emergency medical technicians should examine Medic-Alert™ (Turlock, California) bracelets and should use latex-free gloves when treating a patient with latex allergy. Ideally, the ambulance should carry sterile glass medication vials without rubber stoppers. Lyophilized drugs need to be reconstituted in a glass syringe, not in multidose vials. If these precautions are not taken, the emergency physician will be further exposing a latex-sensitive patient to even more latex antigens.

A comprehensive protocol for the management of latex-allergic patients should be developed for each emergency department. In some hospitals, a latex-free emergency cart has been developed for use throughout the hospital. In the emergency department, the patient should be positioned on a mattress that has no latex mattress cover. A stockinet should always be wrapped around the extremity beneath the blood pressure cuff. Cover the patient's finger with a plastic baggy or Saran

Wrap™ before applying a pulse oximeter. Medications should not be injected through latex IV ports. Covering the latex ports with colored tapes or caps is a helpful warning to hospital personnel.

Management of Type I Allergic Reactions

Antihistamines of the HI class and sympathomimetic agents often provide symptomatic relief for urticaria and angioedema. Cyproheptadine, hydroxyzine, and a combination of H1 and H2 antihistamines are another important therapeutic consideration for treating angioedema and urticaria. Prolonged treatment with topically applied corticosteroids is not recommended in the management of type I allergic reactions.

Antihistamines are the best specific end-organ antagonists for allergic rhinitis. The side effects, which include drowsiness and gastrointestinal distress, following administration of these agents may limit the dosage of the prescribed antihistamine. Topical administration of α-adrenergic agents may be helpful in treating upper respiratory symptoms, but this treatment is accompanied by rebound vasodilatation after prolonged usage.

Because episodes of urticaria, angioedema, rhinitis, and asthma may progress to anaphylaxis, the emergency physician must be prepared to treat this life-threatening condition. Mild initial symptoms may be controlled by the administration of 0.2 mL to 0.5 mL of 1:1000 epinephrine subcutaneously, with repeated doses as required at three-minute intervals. In severe cases, an intravenous infusion should be initiated to provide a route for administration of epinephrine, diluted 1:50,000. If significant hypotension persists, vasopressors, fluids, and volume expanders must also be administered. Oxygen via a nasal catheter may be initially helpful, but endotracheal intubation is mandatory if progressive hypoxia exists. Antihistamines, diphenhydramine (50 mg to 80 mg intramuscularly or intravenously) are valuable for treatment of urticaria, angioedema and bronchospasm, respectively. If persistent bronchospasm and hypotension occurs, intravenous corticosteroids may be useful.

Long-term Management of Latex Allergies

Education about latex avoidance is mandatory in preventing allergic reactions in latex-sensitive patients. The patient must learn the long list of medical and consumer products that contain latex. Patients should be provided with a list of latex-free products for daily or occupational use. They should carry rubber-free examination gloves when seeking medical or dental care. Because there is cross-reactivity between latex and fruit antigens, patients should use care when first consuming these fruits after diagnosis. All latex-allergic patients should wear a Medic-Alert™ bracelet and carry an emergency epinephrine kit at all times.

Latex-Safe Environment

The Task Force on Allergic Reactions to Latex of the American Academy of Allergy and Immunology has recommended that medical procedures performed on latex-sensitive patients should be conducted in a latex-safe environment.[6] A latex-safe environment is one in which no latex gloves are used by any personnel. In addition, there should be no latex accessories (catheters, adhesives, tourniquets, anesthesia equipment, etc.) that come into direct contact with the patient. Detailed perioperative treatment plans should be published for hospital personnel managing latex-sensitive patients. These protocols recommend preoperative prophylactic administration of glucocorticoids and both H1- and H2-class antihistamines to latex-sensitive individuals undergoing surgery.

References Cited in this Appendix

1. Kelly KJ, Kurup VP,, Zacharisen M, Resnick A, and Fink JN. Skin and serologic testing in the diagnosis of latex allergy. *J Allergy Clin Immun.* 1993; 91: 1140-1145.

2. Spaner D, Dolovich J, Tarlo S, Sussman G, Buttoo K. Hypersensitivity to natural latex. *J Allergy Clin Immunol.* 1989;83:1135-1137.

3. Charous BL. The puzzle of latex allergy: some answers, still more questions. *Ann Allergy.* 1994;73:277-281.

4. Kelly KJ, Kurup VP, Reijula KE, Fink JN. The diagnosis of natural rubber latex allergy. *J Allergy Clin Immunol.* 1994; 93:813-816.

5. Heese A, vHintzenstern J, Peters KP, Koch HU, Hornstein OP. Allergic and irritant reactions to rubber gloves in medical health services: spectrum, diagnostic approach, and therapy. *J Am Acad Dermatol,* 1991;25:831-839.

6. Task force on allergic reactions to latex: committee report. *J Allergy Clin Immunol.* 1993;92:16-18.

Latex Avoidance Protocol

Management of a latex-allergic patient in an ambulance, emergency department, and hospital can be very difficult because latex exists everywhere in medical environments. Emergency medical technicians should examine Medic-Alert™ (Turlock, California) bracelets and use latex-free gloves that meet with National Fire Protection Association 1999 Standards when treating a patient with latex allergy. Because all latex gloves contain varying amounts of allergen, the use of latex-free gloves is mandatory. Health professionals must be aware, however, that these latex-free gloves are not as comfortable to wear as latex gloves. Moreover, they are relatively inelastic and more difficult to don than latex gloves. Ideally, the ambulance should carry sterile glass medication vials without rubber stoppers. Drug manipulation should be performed in a glass syringe, not in multidose vials. If these precautions are not taken, the emergency medical technician will further expose a latex-sensitive patient to latex antigens.

Each emergency department must develop a comprehensive protocol for the management of latex-allergic patients.

Checklists help as reminders of the components of a latex-safe hospital. Because it is impossible to resuscitate a patient with a latex allergy using latex equipment, it is particularly important that the emergency department be latex-safe. It is far simpler for the staff to make the entire emergency department latex-safe than it is to maintain separate rooms that are latex-safe. A latex-free emergency cart must be developed for use throughout the emergency department. In the emergency department, the patient should be positioned on a mattress that has no latex mattress cover. A nonlatex, disposable blood pressure cuff should be wrapped around the patients arm. The patient's finger should be wrapped with a plastic baggy or Saran Wrap™ before a pulse oximeter is applied. Medications should not be injected through latex intravenous ports. Many medical centers find that covering the latex ports with colored tapes or caps helps warn hospital personnel. Pharmacies, too, should be latex-safe. All drugs should be in vials without rubber caps, and all medications and intravenous solutions should be prepared under a latex-safe protocol.

The operating room may be one of the most challenging areas to make latex-safe. While it is not possible to totally eliminate all latex from surgery, the operating room should be as latex-free as possible. Gloves with the deadly cornstarch dust and high levels of latex allergen must be banned from the operating room. Eliminating powdered latex gloves dramatically reduces airborne latex particles to very low levels. Powder-free gloves should also contain low levels of chemical irritants as well as latex allergens. While it is relatively safe to use these gloves in patients who are not allergic to latex, they cannot be used in patients with latex allergy or patients in a high-risk group. For these patients, nonlatex gloves are mandatory.

Anesthesia for surgery is probably the single most dangerous threat to the latex-allergic patient. Many of the most serious reactions to latex have occurred during anesthesia. While it is difficult to determine the source of the latex antigen in these patients (e.g., latex mask, anesthesia circuit, drugs, etc.), it is essential that no latex products be used in the delivery of anesthesia to patients with latex allergy or in high-risk groups. Latex-safe precautions should be continued after transfer from the operating room to the recovery room, the intensive care unit, and the patient's room.

The same precautions must be instituted in the delivery suite in obstetrics and gynecology. Many institutions place all newborns on latex-avoidance precautions to prevent the development of a new generation of patients with latex allergy. The risk of developing latex allergy is especially high in children with congenital anomalies or in premature babies who might spend the first weeks or months of their lives in the intensive care nursery. Consequently, nipples and pacifiers must also be latex-free. Because radiology is a site used by all patients, it must be latex-safe and follow latex-safe policies and procedures.

Education on latex avoidance is mandatory to prevent allergic reactions in latex-sensitive patients. The patient must learn the long list of medical and consumer products that contain latex. Patients should be provided with a list of latex-free products for daily or occupational use. They should carry latex-free examination gloves when seeking medical or dental care. Because of the cross-reactivity between latex and fruit antigens, patients should use care when first consuming these fruits after diagnosis. All latex-allergic patients should wear a Medic-Alert™ bracelet and carry an emergency epinephrine kit at all times.

Affected healthcare workers must be reassigned to a latex-free environment. If the worker's degree of allergy endangers personal safety, the hospital must reassign the worker to a latex-free treatment area that treats less critically ill patients.

Healthcare Worker Disability

Healthcare workers with severe persistent allergic symptoms despite avoidance and the use of medications may seek worker's compensation or disability. Ideally, this occupational problem is best solved by the creation of a safe workplace environment for the employee, allowing the employee to continue his or her career after diagnosis of latex allergy. This goal appears attainable, and would not be cost-prohibitive to an educated hospital administration. At present, however, healthcare workers with persistent respiratory symptoms or histories of latex-associated life-threatening allergic reactions may not be able to continue working. Consequently, documentation of the course of the patient's problem, physical examination, positive laboratory tests, and measurements of disability, such as breathing studies (i.e., pulmonary function tests), may be requested. Worker's compensation and disability claims are subject to different criteria and processes from state to state.

Making Your Hospital Latex-Safe

Many prestigious hospitals have established a latex-safe program. Consequently, latex-safe environments have become a standard of care. Health professionals use the term latex-safe because a latex-free environment is nearly impossible to achieve in a hospital setting.

The first step in becoming a latex-safe hospital is to form a committee comprising members from all of the following departments: the Department of Internal Medicine, Department of Surgery, Department of Radiology, Department of Anesthesia, Department of Obstetrics and Gynecology, Department of Nursing, Pharmacy, Respiratory Therapy, Laboratory, Dietary, Housekeeping, Admitting, Department of Home Care, Maintenance, and Administration. This committee would be responsible for developing guidelines, policies, and procedures that ensure the hospital environment is as free of latex as possible. Policies and procedures are needed in the following areas:

Products

- The presence of latex in all nonmedical products (mats, carpets, chairs) used in the hospital must be listed.
- A list of all medical products containing latex must be developed with acceptable nonlatex alternatives.

Equipment

- All emergency carts should be latex-safe.
- Latex-free ventilation equipment should be available.
- Packages for special procedures and surgery must be separately prepared so that they are latex-safe.

Patients

- Admission questionnaires and protocols must be developed and implemented.
- Surgical, obstetric, special procedure, anesthesia, and pharmacy protocols are mandatory.
- General nursing protocols contribute to the establishment of a latex-safe environment.
- Discharge protocols are necessary to ensure appropriate patient follow-up.

Employees

- Latex allergy prevention protocols are necessary to reduce the frequency of sensitization.
- Latex-allergic employee protocols are required to allow the employee to work in a latex-safe environment.

Education

- An educational program must be instituted to all members of the hospital regarding the importance of a latex-free environment.

Guide for Malpractice and Consumer Product Litigation

The physician, nurse, hospital, and manufacturer are all potentially liable for injuries sustained by the patient by the use of a particular product during medical treatment. To succeed in such a claim, the patient must demonstrate, among other things, that the product caused his/her injury. A healthcare employee who develops a work-related disability may have a claim for worker's compensation. In addition, depending on the nature of the disability, certain accommodations may be necessary in the workplace if the employee is to continue performing his or her job.

What do these two situations have in common? Both the patient and the employee may have a potential claim. Neither may be able to settle their claims and damages voluntarily. Both may require the services of a lawyer. Neither is likely to have had contact with a lawyer in the past. Choosing a lawyer is an important decision. For persons injured as a result of medically related treatment or employment, this fact may be particularly true because the injury may be complex. In some ways, choosing a lawyer is like planting a garden. Lawyers may differ in yield and quality of results. Some lawyers will meet or exceed a client's expectations and will produce as they promise. Others may not produce what they promise or not produce at all. Having the right lawyer for your needs is important.

When to See a Lawyer

If you have been treated by a healthcare provider and, as a result of the care, subsequently develop additional injuries you may have a claim for damages. One example is the development of postoperative adhesions. As discussed below, this complication may not be the result of malpractice or a defective product. Healthcare providers are not guarantors of a positive outcome. However, if you develop complications that can be traced directly to the treatment you received, it may be appropriate to seek advice from a lawyer.

A healthcare worker who develops a work-related condition, such as a latex allergy, may require accommodations at work to continue employment. This accomodation could range from the use of alternative surgical or examination gloves to a transfer to a department that minimizes exposure to the product. Often employers willingly cooperate with an employee to explore alternatives. In such cases, it may not be necessary to seek assistance from a lawyer.

Discussing a potential claim with a lawyer does not mean you are required to litigate, or even retain the lawyer after the initial conference. In some instances, a lawyer will conclude after discussion with you and a review of available information, that there is no basis for pursuing the matter. In other instances, while a potential claim may exist, you may be advised the time and expense may not justify pursuing the matter. Finally, it may be possible to settle the issue with the healthcare provider or hospital without resorting to litigation. Seeking legal advice is a step in determining your options. It will enable you to make an informed decision about whether to pursue a claim and the likely results.

Selecting a Lawyer

Once you have decided to seek assistance from a lawyer, the next step is selecting the lawyer. Most often, people select a lawyer based on the recommendation of a friend or family member. Some state or local Bar Associations operate a referral service that can refer you to a lawyer in your area who handles cases similar to yours. None of these methods guarantees that the lawyer you contact will be capable of handling your case. Even if competent to handle your case, the lawyer may not be a person with whom you are comfortable.

The person seeking assistance from a lawyer must do some homework to select the correct lawyer. Because litigation can be a time-consuming process and may involve inquiry into the most intimate details of your life, it is important for you to be comfortable with the lawyer you select. Your lawyer will become part of your life, and you must believe the lawyer will protect your privacy and listen to your concerns. The lawyer may review your entire medical and employment history, inquire about your personal life and relationships, and delve into many aspects of your daily life. You must be able to trust your lawyer, so pay attention to your feelings about the lawyer when you initially meet.

You start by making an appointment with the lawyer for an initial consultation. The appointment is the time to get as much information as possible so you can make an informed decision about whether to hire this lawyer. Do not be afraid to ask questions. Prepare a list of questions ahead of time. Ask the lawyer about his or her experience with similar cases. Has the lawyer sued hospitals or healthcare practitioners for malpractice in the past? Has the lawyer had experience with claims under the Americans With Disabilities Act? Have any of these cases been tried? Does the lawyer consult with other lawyers who are experienced in such cases? Is the lawyer a member of any professional trial lawyers' group? Is the lawyer certified as an expert in your type of case? A good lawyer will be honest and tell you when he or she does not have all the answers. If the lawyer cannot answer your questions or cannot handle your case, you should ask the lawyer for the names of other lawyers with experience in handling this kind of case.

You may want to ask the lawyer if he or she also represents hospitals or healthcare professionals. Particularly in smaller communities, lawyers may do work for local healthcare professionals. Do not be surprised if the lawyer asks you for the names of the people involved. These questions are necessary because it might be a conflict of interest for the lawyer to represent you against someone the lawyer already represents. Just because a lawyer does work for hospitals or healthcare professionals does not mean the lawyer cannot represent you fairly. Sometimes this can be an advantage because his or her prior representation in the field gives the lawyer a broader experience base. It is, however, something you should discuss seriously with the lawyer to assess his or her attitude about representing your side of the case.

The Cost of Legal Services

You should always discuss with a lawyer what charges you will incur for his/her services. The two most common fee arrangements are hourly rates and contingency fees. Under an hourly rate arrangement, the lawyer will bill you for the amount of time spent based on a stated hourly rate. You will also be expected to pay for out-of-pocket costs advanced by the lawyer such as postage, long-distance telephone charges, photocopies, and filing fees.

Under the contingency fee method, you agree to compensate the lawyer for costs and time spent based on a percentage of any amounts paid to you. This method is generally used in personal injury, medical malpractice, and worker's compensation cases. In each case, you may be asked to pay in advance an amount of money, called a retainer, before work begins on your case. The retainer fee pays for at least some of the costs and services.

Ask the lawyer to explain the fee arrangements in detail. If the agreement is for an hourly rate, ask the lawyer to tell you the applicable rates for all lawyers who will work on your case. Ask how often you will receive a bill, and what detail or information will be on the bill. If the agreement is for a contingency fee, ask the lawyer to explain the terms and percentages that will be used to establish the fee. Remember, you are the consumer, and the retention of a lawyer is in large measure a business transaction. Do not be afraid to ask the lawyer to prepare a written fee agreement, spelling out the terms and conditions of the retainer. A written agreement is the only way to avoid most future misunderstandings about what you will be charged.

What You Can Expect from a Lawyer

Lawyers do not have a crystal ball that will predict precisely what will happen in your case. Their opinion about your case will necessarily become clearer as the facts become clearer. Gathering facts is part of the process of providing competent representation. Lawyers also do not have a magic wand that will give you instant results or an immediate recovery. Lawyers do have the skills to handle investigation, research, paperwork, negotiation, discovery, and litigation. A lawyer should be expected to be familiar with all of the legal procedures necessary to pursue your claim. He or she should have a working knowledge of applicable legal concepts. A lawyer will also know the courtroom procedures and rules applicable to your situation. Often, lawyers can also serve as a resource on where to look for assistance.

Fundamentally, lawyers are problem-solvers. Part of a lawyer's livelihood is working out problems through negotiation. People hire lawyers because of the lawyer's skill, experience, and judgment. As facts develop in a case and additional information is gathered, you should expect your lawyer to advise you of the effect of any new information. You can and should demand certain additional things from your lawyer. The lawyer should return your phone calls. The lawyer should send you copies of correspondence and other legal documents pertaining to your case and keep you informed of any progress. In general, the lawyer should not make any agreements or commitments on your behalf without consulting you first. Some matters, such as agreeing to dates and times when lawyers must meet, will occur without discussing the matter with you. This occurrence is, however, an exception. Your lawyer should also keep you regularly informed of the work performed and, if you are being billed at an hourly rate or for costs, he or she should regularly bill you for the work or costs, preferably monthly.

What a Lawyer Can Expect from You

While this appendix has emphasized what to look for in a lawyer you can trust, trust must run both ways. A lawyer cannot help you unless you also follow certain rules. When going to meet a lawyer, you should take with you all available papers about your situation. When setting up the initial appointment, ask the lawyer whether there are any documents or records you should bring with you. You need to be honest with your lawyer. If you cannot do that, you might as well not hire a lawyer because he or she cannot effectively represent you without all information. Do not hold back because you think it may not be important or because it may embarrass you. Let the lawyer decide whether the information is important or relevant.

Listen carefully to your lawyer's assessment of your case. You may bring to a meeting certain expectations or opinions about the value of your case. The purpose of retaining a lawyer is to procure his or her professional opinion about the value of your case. This opinion will not always mirror your own. The lawyer's job becomes doubly difficult if the client's expectations are unwarrantedly optimistic, while the opposing side takes the most pessimistic approach.

Fundamental Legal Concepts

If you are thinking about hiring a lawyer, you probably have a number of questions. Are the powders on the gloves used by healthcare professionals safe? Have people developed health problems that may be attributed to glove powders? Are healthcare workers who develop health problems attributable to gloves or glove powders entitled to request accommodation at their place of employment? Is a person whose injuries are caused by gloves or powder entitled to compensation? If so, from whom? These and other questions are designed to develop sources of litigation. Litigation is extremely time-consuming. It can also be financially and emotionally costly. For these reasons, it is important to be prepared when retaining counsel.

Generally, there are three types of claims that may be asserted when dealing with injuries related to powder. The basic elements of each type of claim and examples will be discussed below. The following discussion is general in nature because the facts may affect the analysis. Further, state law may limit or modify the general rules. No attempt is made to survey all the variations that may exist in state law. If an injured plaintiff can establish that his injury or her injury was caused by a specific product used in the operating room, the manufacturer and product distributors, the surgeon, the hospital, and any other healthcare provider involved could be potentially liable for damages. Such liability may include claims for both medical malpractice and product liability. Lawyers refer to both types of claims generally as "torts." The law of torts is a method of making adjustment between parties for conflicting claims for damages. Some of the earliest appearances of the claim of negligence in modern times were against persons who held themselves out as being competent in positions of direct service to the public, such as surgeons. The theory was that these individuals held themselves out to the public as persons in whom faith and confidence could repose and, therefore, they assumed a duty to provide proper service. If they breached that duty, they should be held liable for any damage suffered.

Medical Malpractice

In treating a person, a healthcare professional is generally required to use the degree of care, skill, and judgment usually exercised in the same or similar circumstances by the average healthcare professional. This standard takes into account the state of medical science at the time the patient was treated. A person asserting a claim for malpractice must prove the healthcare professional failed to conform to this standard. A physician does not guarantee the results of his care and treatment. Rather, a physician must use reasonable care. A physician, for example, cannot be found negligent simply because a bad result may have followed from the care and treatment he or she rendered. Medicine is not an exact science. Therefore, the issue in a malpractice case is whether the physician failed to use the degree of care, skill, and judgment exercised by the average physician. The degree of care, skill, and judgment that is usually exercised by a doctor is not a matter within the common knowledge of laypersons. For that reason, experts are normally used to explain these standards.

A second important element in any malpractice claim is causation. The cause question asks whether there was a causal connection between negligence on the part of the physician and the patient's injury. A person's negligence is a cause of an injury if the negligence was a substantial factor in producing the present condition of the plaintiff's health. This question does not ask about "the cause," but rather about "a cause." The reason is that there can be more than one cause of an injury. The negligence of one or more persons can cause an injury. An injury can also be the result of the natural progression of an injury.

For example, if you have a history of postoperative adhesions or a known sensitivity to latex, and the physician uses a powdered latex glove, this action may be negligent. If you later develop complications, such as an obstruction, granuloma, or adhesion provoked by glove powder, it can be said the injury was caused by the use of the powdered latex gloves. Confirmation of the cause generally requires pathological examination to verify that the cause was a foreign body (e.g., powder), rather than unavoidable trauma or infection.

Product Liability

Product liability is a subspecies of negligence. As discussed, infra, it has been asserted as a basis for recovery against glove manufacturers in the past. This theory of liability is designed to provide recovery from a manufacturer or supplier for injury caused by defects in products. Product liability is a rapidly changing area and varies greatly from state to state. The duty of a manufacturer or supplier of a product is to exercise ordinary care in ensuring that the product will not create an unreasonable risk of injury or damage to the user or owner when used in its intended or foreseeable manner.[1] This duty may be, ". . . approached from the standpoint of the standard of care to be exercised by the reasonably prudent person in the shoes of the defendant manufacturer or supplier."[2] A manufacturer, among other requirements, is required to exercise ordinary care in the manufacture of its product in the following aspects: (1) safe design of the product so that it will be fit for its intended or foreseeable purpose; (2) construction of the product so that the materials and workmanship furnished will render the product safe for its intended or foreseeable use; (3) adequate inspections and tests to determine the extent of defects as to both materials and workmanship; and (4) adequate warnings of danger in the use of the product and adequate instructions as to the proper use of the product, which is dangerous, when used as intended.[3]

A warning or instruction, when required, must be reasonably calculated to reach and to be understood by those likely to use the product. The warning must be sufficient to inform the average user of the nature and extent of the danger that he or she may encounter in the use of the product.[4] The packaging used for surgical or examination gloves contains warnings or cautionary statements. These statements advise the wearer of hazards associated with powder and recommend removal of the powder before use. Advertising for powder-free gloves often includes reference to the advantages of such gloves, including reduction of the risk of powder-related postoperative complications, such as adhesion-formation. These warnings, coupled with the growing body of medical literature on powder-related complications, are an indication of the developing acknowledgement that powder presents a danger.

In some circumstances, the warnings may shield the manufacturer from liability if it is sufficient to warn the healthcare provider of the dangers associated with powder. However, the warnings may not be sufficient to shield the healthcare provider from liability for medical malpractice if appropriate steps were not taken in accordance with the warnings. The warning may also create potential problems for the healthcare provider if a less dangerous alternative was available for a patient at increased risk of complications. For example, if a surgeon has a patient who previously developed postoperative granulomas from glove powder, the use of a powder-free glove is a more appropriate alternative to reduce the risk of such complications.

Before a manufacturer can be held responsible for failure to warn users, it must have actual or constructive notice of the dangers of the product.[5] Where a manufacturer undertakes to give instructions about the proper use of a product, it assumes the duty of providing adequate instructions and calling attention to the dangers to be avoided.[6] In establishing a cause of action for product liability, the plaintiff must show the product was defective, unreasonably dangerous, or somehow foreseeably deleterious to the plaintiff at the time the product left the manufacturers or suppliers hands. The plaintiff must also demonstrate that he or she sustained an injury and that the product's defect or danger was the proximate cause of the injury or damage.

Prior Powder Litigation

Early claims involving glove powders were generally unsuccessful. For example, in 1981, a plaintiff sued a glove manufacturer, alleging the gloves used by her surgeon were defective. She alleged the powder from the gloves caused her to suffer a severe reaction that ultimately required a hysterectomy. The court held the powder used in the manufacturing process in the late 1970s was consistent with the highest degree of quality control and available technology at that time. For that reason, the gloves were held not defective and the claim was dismissed.[7]

Similarly, a plaintiff suing a hospital and glove manufacturer was also unsuccessful in asserting a claim in 1976. The plaintiff in this case had multiple surgeries. Following surgery, the plaintiff developed extensive adhesions and bowel obstruction. The jury found the gloves were unreasonably dangerous, thus meeting one of the required elements for a product liability claim. However, the claim was dismissed because the plaintiff could not prove the obstructions or adhesions were caused by starch from the gloves used in the most recent surgery. This plaintiff had a series of earlier operations; the condition could have been caused by powder from one of the prior surgeries. Thus, although the jury found the gloves unreasonably dangerous, the plaintiff could not demonstrate the injuries were caused by the gloves used at the hospital.[8]

A Massachusetts jury held a glove manufacturer, a gynecologist, and hospital personnel liable for the development of "cornstarch peritonitis" in a case involving a patient who developed intestinal blockage following gynecological surgery.[9] A series of additional cases have been brought against healthcare professionals, hospitals, and manufacturers alleging injury as a result of glove powder. To date, there have been no reported decisions.

In many instances, however, the matter has been settled out of court, and the amount of settlement is not public.

As the cases develop, certain questions appear to affect the outcome. First, is it possible through pathology reports to confirm the presence of glove powder? Second, has a physical injury, such as an adhesion or granuloma, formed as a result of the glove powder? Third, can the presence of the glove powder be traced to a particular operation or manufacturer? Fourth, were protocols and standards of care followed in removing glove powder? A recognition that surgeons could and should be aware of the danger of starch powder seems to be gaining acceptance because of increasing discussion of the subject in medical literature.

Employment-related Issues

In 1990, the U.S. Congress adopted the Americans with Disabilities Act of 1990.[10] The act recognized that a substantial number of Americans have one or more physical disabilities and, as a result, may face discrimination or barriers in employment. The act was intended to establish standards to address discrimination against individuals with disabilities.[11] The act prohibits employers from discriminating against a qualified individual with a disability because of the disability. Discrimination is defined to include a failure to make "reasonable accommodations" to the known physical limitations of an otherwise qualified individual.[12] It also includes the denial of employment opportunities to an applicant or employee, who is otherwise qualified, if the denial is based on the need to make reasonable accommodation to the physical impairments of the person.[13] While there are exceptions to these provisions, the exceptions generally require either a showing of undue hardship or involve a determination of whether an accommodation is "reasonable."

In general, "reasonable accommodations" may include job restructuring, modified work schedules, reassignment to a vacant position, acquisition or modification of equipment or devices, or modification of facilities.[14] The act also contains a brief definition of "undue hardship."[15] These definitions, however, do not address every situation. They are intended to provide guidance. The determination whether an accommodation is "reasonable" or would present an "undue hardship" must be determined on a case-by-case basis.

The physical condition must be a "permanent" condition to qualify as a disability. For example, a temporary back sprain or inability to work for a period of weeks after surgery is a transitory condition and does not qualify as a disability.[16] Additionally, the impairment must substantially limit or impair a major life activity. For example, an employee subject to a lifting restriction because of carpal tunnel syndrome would not be considered disabled if the restriction did not impair performance of his or her job or limit his/her employment opportunities provided the employer did not regard the limitation as a disability.[17]

Assuming an employee is permanently disabled, the next inquiry is whether some type of accommodation is possible or required. This situation generally requires a careful examination of the person's job duties. Are each of the tasks performed by the person "essential" to the job? For example, if the employee is subject to weight limitations, does the job require lifting? If so, is there a similar position available that falls within the weight limitations? If so, reasonable accommodation by reassigning the employee to that position may be required.[18] If no such position is available, however, there is no requirement for a position to be created.

To date there are no reported decisions concerning disabilities related to powder. Claims have been asserted and are pending at this time. Whether any of the claims will be successful is an open question. The answer will depend on a variety of questions. Is the condition complained of a "disability"? Does it limit or impair a major life activity? Does it interfere with the person's ability to perform essential job functions? Are reasonable accommodations possible?

When presented with these issues, the employees should carefully consider these questions. The next step is to determine what job requirements would have to be modified to permit the employee to continue performing his or her job. A common modification used to accommodate powder- or latex-sensitive healthcare workers is the use of powder-free or nonlatex gloves. One study estimated that 7.4 percent of surgeons and 5.6 percent of operating nurses are latex-sensitive.[19] Current research suggests the possibility that glove powder may become airborne and affect persons not directly in contact with powdered latex gloves. Additional research indicates latex-sensitive individuals are able to return to work when coworkers use powder-free latex gloves.[20] In such a situation, the use of powder-free gloves by all persons in the room might need to be considered as a possible accommodation.

The question will be whether such an accommodation is reasonable. If modification is not possible, does another open position exist for which the employee is qualified? Based on the incidence of latex sensitivity in healthcare workers, these are questions likely to be faced with increasing frequency. These questions should be explored with the employer. If the employer is unwilling to discuss the issues, it may be appropriate to seek the advice of an attorney.

References

1. *Smith v. Atco Co.*, 6 Wis. 2d 371, 94 N.W.2d 697 (1959); Restatement, Second, Torts § 395 (1965) Prosser, *Law of Torts* (3d), 648-650 (1964).
2. *Smith v. Atco Co., supra* note 1.
3. *Schwalbach v. Antigo Elec. & Gas Co., 27 Wis.2d 651, 135 N.W.2d 263 (1965);* Smith v. Atco., 266 Wis. 630, 64N.W.2d

226 (1954); *Marsh Wood Products Co. v. babcock & Wilcox Co., supra* note 6; Flies v. Fox Bros. Buick Co., 196 Wis. 196, 218 N.W. 855 (1928); 1 Frumer and Friedman, *Product Liability* § 6.8 (1966); Restatement, Second, Torts (395 (1965); 6 A.L.R.3d 91 (1966).

4. Harper and James, 2 *Law of Torts* § 28.7 at 1548-1549 (1956).
5. *Strahlensorf v. Walgreen Co.,* 16 Wis. 2d 421, 114 N.W.2d 326 (1962); Restatement, *supra* note 20, § 401 at 339 (1965).
6. *Karsteadt v. Phillip Gross H. & S. Co.,* 179 Wis. 110, 190 N.W. 844 (1922).
7. *Flagg v. Dart Industries, Inc.,* U.S. Dist. Ct., Boston, Mass., No. 773833-S, February 1981, 18 Verdict Reporter 114 (Sept. 15, 1981).
8. *Simms v. Southwest Texas Methodist Hospital,* 535 S.W.2d 192 (Tex. App. 1976).
9. *Kohn v. Dart Industries,* U.S. Dist. Ct., D. Mass., No. 73-2051-M, December 1, 1977, 21 ATLA Law Reporter 233 (June 1978).
10. 42 U.S.C. §§ 12101 et seq.
11. 42 U.S.C. § 12101(b).
12. 42 U.S.C. § 12112(b)(5)(A).
13. 42 U.S.C. § 12112(b)(5)(B).
14. 24 U.S.C. §12111(9).
15. 42 U.S.C. § 12111(10).
16. *Presutti v. Felton Brush,* 11 ADD 684, 4 AD Cas. 1511 (DC NH, 1995); *McDonald v. Department of Public Welfare, Polk Ctr.,* 62 F.3d 92 (3rd Cir. 1995).
17. *Fink v. Kitzman,* 881 F.Supp. 1347 (ND Iowa, 1995).
18. *Hunt-Golliday v. Metropolitan Water Reclamation Dist.,* 7 ADD 941 (ND, Ill. 1994).
19. Turjanmaa K. Incidence of immediate allergy to latex gloves in hospital personnel. *Contact Dermatitis* 1987;17:270-275.
20. Tarlo SM, Sussman G, Contala A, Swanson MC. Control of airborne latex by use of powder-free gloves. *J Allergy Clin Immunol.* 1994;93:985-989.

Commercially Available Powder-Free Gloves

TABLE F-1 *Natural Latex Powder-free Examination Gloves*

Supplier	Brand	Lot #	Lowry with Precipitation (μg/g)	LEAP (μg/g)
Microflex	Ultra one	Not Available	< 20	< 0.2
Supertex	Supertex	Not Available	21	< 0.2
Regent	Biogel D	93035	< 20	< 0.2
Aladan	Neutraderm	1081433H	< 20	< 0.2
Phenix Research Products	Bio-Flex Powder-free Exam	Not Available	38	0.3
American Medical Products	Arista Pro Touch	Not Available	24	0.4
Thailand (unknown)	Exam	Not Available	< 20	0.5
Universal	Maytex	Not Available	< 20	0.6
SJS	SJS	9211003	21	0.6
Wembley	Wembley S&N	Not Available	< 20	0.6
Mala Intertrade	Scan Med	Not Available	< 20	0.8
Smith and Nephew Perry	DermaClean X-AM	5766203 800447	< 20	0.8

(continued)

TABLE F-1   *Natural Latex Powder-free Examination Gloves (continued)*

Supplier	Brand	Lot #	Lowry with Precipitation (µg/g)	LEAP (µg/g)
SJS	SJS	Not Available	45	1.1
MRY	MRY	Not Available	< 20	1.3
Thailand (unknown)	Exam	Not Available	< 20	1.3
Microflex	Diamond Grip	Not Available	< 20	1.5
TK Glove	Bodyguard	9310283013	< 20	1.7
Bio-Flex Dental	Bio-Flex Gel	Not Available	< 20	1.9
Marsin	Exam	Not Available	< 20	2.0
Glove India	GAC	Not Available	< 20	2.1
Premier	Premier	Not Available	< 20	2.1
China (unknown)	Exam	Not Available	< 20	2.2
Molnyche	Molnyche	Not Available	< 20	3.8
SJS/American Health Products	Glove Tex	Not Available	51	6.5
Malaysia (unknown)	Exam	Not Available	93	6.9
Marsin	Exam	Not Available	75	9.3
Sime Group	Sime Darby	Not Available	75	14
Crosstex	Crosstex	Not Available	92	14
IBM	CR10	000022	21	15
Safeskin	PowderFree	11A4053BC	33	19
Malaysia (unknown)	Exam	Not Available	82	79
PT Surya Milani	PAC	Not Available	829	82
Steriltex	Sterigel	Not Available	516	92
China (unknown)	Exam	Not Available	1089	578

Source: *OR Manager. 1995;11(6);4. Copyright 1995, OR Manager.*

TABLE F-2 *Natural Latex Powder-free Surgical Gloves*

Supplier	Brand	Lot #	Lowry with Precipitation (µg/g)	LEAP (µg/g)
Regent	Biogel M	943013	< 20	< 0.2
Johnson & Johnson	Ultralon	13831321629	108	0.2
Ansell	Ansell	312520104	47	0.4
Fuji Latex	Pristine	4070989	32	0.5
Baxter	Triflex	K4E042	< 20	0.6
Regent	Biogel	944120	< 20	0.6
Fuji Latex	Surgeon-Plus	4090389	20	0.9
Fuji Latex	Pristine XTRA	4150389	34	0.9
Baxter	Ultrafree	K4B014	< 20	1.3
Becton Dickinson	Dextren	02072328F	33	3.4
SmartCare	Royal Shield	920828	49	6.8
Ansell Medical	Nutex	402556404	36	8.2
Smith +Nephew Perry	Encore	729615B	50	21

Source: *OR Manager. 1995;11(6);6. Copyright 1995, OR Manager.*

TABLE F-3 *Protein Levels of Common Surgical Gloves**

Glove Name	Lot #	Lowry with Precipitation (µg/g)	LEAP (µg/g)
Powdered			
Triflex	PGS-5E335	61	12.3
Baxter	PGS-5E349		
Microtouch	PO2528	333	51
J&J	AO20666		
Hypoallergenic			
Neutralon	602529	192	48.9
J&J	602730		
Ultraderm	PGS-4P025	69	13.1
Baxter	PGS5B081		

(continued)

TABLE F-3 *Protein Levels of Common Surgical Gloves (continued)*

Glove Name	Lot #	Lowry with Precipitation (µg/g)	LEAP (µg/g)
Eudermic	02075009K	< 28	5.9
Maxxim	02074290U		
Powder-free			
Biogel	9500384	< 28	< 0.5
Regent	9500138		
Biogel M	944158	< 28	< 0.2
Regent	94403		
Encore	736732N	130	18.4
Ansell/Perry	736723N		
Supra	01A434A	< 28	4.4
Safeskin	A42856355A		
Ultrafree	3D7132	< 28	1.8
Baxter	3D7134		
Dextran Clear	02074210	< 28	3.1
Maxxim	02075100		
Orthopedic			
Maxxus	E03062	439	115
J&J	10231312611		
Ortho	742914W	357	89.4
Ansell/Perry	739483		

*Gloves from two different lot numbers were collected in 1995 and tested using ASTM D5712 modified Lowry and the LEAP ELISA assay (Donald H. Beezhold, Ph.D.).

Directory of Testing, Standards and Regulatory Agencies

Safety Equipment Institute
1901 North Moore Street
Suite 808
Arlington, VA 22209
Telephone (703) 525-3354
Fax (703) 525-2148

Inchcape Testing Services NA Inc.
ETL Testing Laboratories, Inc.
3933 US Route 11
Cortland, NY 13045
Telephone (607) 753-6711
Fax (607) 756-6711

U.S. Department of Health and
Human Services
Public Health Services
Food and Drug Administration
Division of Small Manufacturers
Assistance (DSMA)

5600 Fishers Lane
Rockville, MD 20857
Telephone (301) 443-6597
Fax (301) 443-8818

National Fire Protection
Association (NFPA)
1 Batterymarch Park
P.O. Box 9101
Quincy, MA 02269-9101
Telephone 1-800 344-3555

Underwriters Laboratory
12 Laboratory Dr.
P.O. Box 13995
Research Triangle Park, NC
27709-3995
Telephone (919) 549-1400
Fax (919) 549-1842

Association for the Advancement of Medical Instrumentation
3330 Washington Blvd.
Suite 400
Arlington, VA 22201
Telephone 1-800-332-2264

North American Science Associates, Inc.
2261 Tracy Rd
Northwood, OH 43619
Telephone: (419) 666-2954
Fax: (419) 666-2954

ASTM Standards for Glove Testing

ASTM Designation: D 412-92
Standard Test Methods for Vulcanized Rubber and Thermoplastic Rubbers and Thermoplastic Elastomers-Tensions

ASTM Designation: D 4157-92
Standard Test Method for Abrasion Resistance of Textile Fabrics (Oscillatory Cylinder Method)

ASTM Designation: F 392-93
Standard Test Method for Flex Durability of Flexible Barrier Materials

ASTM Designation: D 573-88 (Re-approved 1994)
Standard Test Method for Rubber-Deterioration in an Air Oven

ASTM Designation: F 1342-91 (Re-approved 1996)
Standard Test Method for Protective Clothing Material Resistance to Puncture

ASTM Designation: D 3577-91
Standard Specifications for Rubber Surgical Gloves

ASTM Designation: D 3578-95
Standard Specification for Rubber Examination Gloves

ASTM Designation: D 5151-92
Standard Test Method for Detection of Holes in Medical Gloves

ASTM Designation: D1003-95
Standard Test Method for Haze and Luminous Transmittance of Transparent Plastic

ASTM Designation: F134-85
Standard Test Method for Determining Hermeticity of Electron Devices with a Helium Mass Spectrometer Leak Detector

ASTM Designation: F1359-91
Determining the Liquid-Tight Integrity of Chemical Protective Suits or Ensembles Under Static Conditions

ASTM Designation: F 903-96
Standard Test Methods for Resistance of Materials Used in Protective Clothing to Penetration by Liquids

ASTM Designation: D5712-95
Standard Test Method for Analysis of Protein in Natural Rubber and Its Products

Index